AGGRESSION
A Nurses' Guide to Therapeutic Management

AGGRESSION

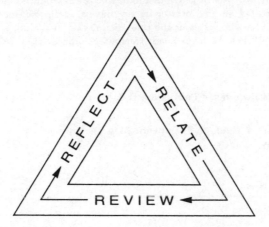

A Nurses' Guide to Therapeutic Management

Gerald A. Farrell MSc RMN RGN DipN(Lond) CertEd
Colin Gray BA(Hons) RMN RGN DipN(Lond) CertEd

Scutari Press
London

Scutari Press is a division of Scutari Projects Ltd,
the publishing company of the Royal College of Nursing

First published in 1992

British Library Cataloguing in Publication Data

Farrell, Gerald A.
  Aggression: Nurses' Guide to Therapeutic Management
  I. Title II. Gray, Colin
  610.73

ISBN 1–871364–60–4

Typeset by J&L Composition Ltd, Filey, North Yorkshire
Printed and bound in Great Britain by
Biddles Ltd, Guildford and King's Lynn

The Authors

Gerald A. Farrell MSc RMN RGN DipN(Lond) CertEd
Lecturer
School of Nursing
Edith Cowan University
Churchlands
Western Australia

Colin Gray BA(Hons) RMN RGN DipN(Lond) CertEd
Nurse Tutor
Avon and Gloucestershire College of Health
Gloucester

Line Drawings:

Adrian Bradshaw-Jones BA(Hons) RMN
Littlemore Hospital
Oxford

Contents

From GF

To Hiong, Lee-Ann and Jon-Lee.
My best teachers yet.

From CG

To JSD. For some reason.

Acknowledgements

The authors are grateful to all their colleagues at Littlemore Hospital, Oxford, who read early drafts and gave encouragement. Tim Woodward, especially, made several valuable suggestions for modifications. Thanks are also due to Robin Snowball, librarian at the Cairns Library, Radcliffe Infirmary, for his patience and insight. Also, our appreciation of the team at Scutari and their reviewers must be noted.

Finally, we are deeply indebted to Dr Jeffrey Garland, Principal Clinical Psychologist in the Department of Psychology, Warneford Hospital, Oxford. His enthusiasm and support in the early days of the project convinced us that our efforts would be worthwhile.

GF
CG

Preface

It is probable that most people who contemplate a nursing career give little thought to being involved in aggressive incidents. Yet a moment's reflection on everyday relationships highlights aggression, whether it be an elbow in the bus queue or a hurtful remark – both fairly common experiences. It would be surprising, therefore, if patients were not sometimes angry and aggressive, considering their added stress of being ill in an alien environment, and it would be naïve to think that nurses do not get angry from time to time: looking after someone else can be demanding and stressful.

Aggressive behaviour itself is invariably unpleasant, and to be involved in it typically unsettles those to whom it is unfamiliar. Paradoxically, it demands the most careful and expert responses at a time when one is far from being composed. We believe that for a nurse to be therapeutic in the face of patients' aggressive behaviour requires expert knowledge in the management of aggression, but this knowledge cannot be obtained without first gaining a deep understanding of aggression itself. Furthermore, the most refined skills are seen in nurses who are aware of their own feelings about aggression and who can acknowledge the anger they themselves sometimes feel. Our aim in writing this guide is to help nurses' personal development: understanding aggression, increasing their knowledge of management and heightening their awareness of feelings about aggression. Those in other caring roles will find the information equally useful.

The notion underlying the organisation of this book is that aggression is best dealt with by moving through a three-stage cycle. The first part, REFLECT, requires the nurse to develop a full understanding of aggression in its context. The roles of self and other people and the physical elements of the environment are considered. The second section, RELATE, explores the parts that can be played by direct interpersonal interventions (both verbal and physical) in managing aggression. The need for prevention and anticipation of aggression is emphasised, and we show how this can be achieved by environmental manipulation and the use of interpersonal skills. We believe that most incidents of aggression can be either avoided altogether or contained without recourse to physical force. However, the need for physical intervention as an unavoidable last resort is not over-looked. Part III, REVIEW, looks at the processes that should follow an aggressive incident – measures that can help everyone to gain from the experience of aggression and that can prevent future aggression. Throughout these three stages, ideas, sugges-tions and techniques that are theory-based and practical are brought together. Finally, in the Appendix there is a digest of steps for the prevention of aggression.

All the ideas and guidance in this book are the result of many years of practising and teaching therapeutic approaches to aggressive patients, both in psychiatry and in general settings. A short text such as this does not do justice to that experience, but inevitably the discussion must be limited by the space available. Especially difficult was knowing when to include detailed guidance applicable to a few situations and when to opt for more global suggestions, which might be applied to many situations. We hope that we have achieved the right balance.

HOW TO USE THE GUIDE

It could be said that the development of expertise in the management of aggression requires three things: knowledge, self-understanding and practical experience. This book is designed to improve knowledge and understanding as well as to offer pointers for action in the practical situation.

Although the guide is an important resource that can be used by individuals, some readers will achieve greater benefit if its use is followed by group work of some kind. It is not intended to be a definitive cookbook of aggression management, with a recipe for every encounter; the reader *must* be prepared to evaluate suggestions and apply them, and most people will find this more valuable as a group exercise.

Much can also be gained if the underlying principles are tried out and refined during everyday relationships, for example with friends and partners, as these can, from time to time, involve angry exchanges. Furthermore, we suggest that the student should look out for examples of aggression management in the community. Apart from those in colleagues, the authors have found role models in the parent dealing with an angry child in the supermarket and the bus conductor jollying along a drunk.

Much of this material can be used by team leaders as the basis for a teaching programme at unit level. One of the difficulties of learning new skills from books is that people can feel awkward without a suitable context, so it is hoped that group settings will enable readers to adapt and shape the ideas and guidelines for their own work settings and their own styles of interaction. However, the case studies, especially, are geared to individual study, and exercises are included to provoke thought. These *should* be completed alone and then, ideally, responses should be compared with those of colleagues.

One area which certainly *must not* be self-taught is that of physical intervention. An experienced instructor is essential for its safe learning as many of the breakaway techniques, for example, could put the nurse at risk if not carried out successfully.

What all these learning strategies have in common for their success is a commitment to a continuing cycle of practice, review and planning for similar problems – and then more practice. The unique nature of each aggressive encounter ensures that there will always be something new to learn.

GF
CG
Oxford, January 1992

Glossary

In literature on aggression, the same terms are used in different ways. The aim of this glossary is to clarify the meanings as used in this text.

Abuse To speak harshly or coarsely to another; to disparage another.

Adult One of the three ego states in transactional analysis. The other two ego states are the child ego state and the parent ego state; together they are said to form the personality.

Aggression Refers to aggressive behaviour. This is defined as the infliction of harm or injury (either physical or psychological) upon another. This definition includes placing another under threat of harm or injury.

Assault A violent attack by either words, physical means or both. In the legal sense, it refers to reasonable fear or apprehension of the unjustified use of force.

Assertion Assertive people acknowledge their own self-worth and recognise the worth of others. Assertive people are neither passive, aggressive nor manipulative. They stand up for their rights and express their views calmly and directly.

Breakaway techniques Includes a range of methods to effect escape from an aggressor. However, many of the methods should only be attempted after training by a facilitator experienced in such techniques.

Child One of the three ego states in transactional analysis. It has two forms: the adapted child and the natural child.

Counselling A general term referring to attempts to help another live as effective a life as possible. It is often employed for personal, marital, sexual and occupational difficulties. It is not to be confused with advice-giving.

Hostile Unfriendly towards another, with malevolent intent. It may also refer to an environment, as in a hostile or forbidding place.

Hostility   A state of tension between two or more people or groups.

Interpersonal   Referring to verbal and non-verbal communication between two or more people.

Interpersonal skills   The verbal and non-verbal skills required for effective social intercourse. The term implies that communication skills can be learned and refined in the same way as other skills. Similar terms are 'social skills', 'face-to-face interaction' and 'people skills'.

Intrapersonal   Refers to our internal thoughts and feelings. It is used to refer to the subjective observations we have of ourselves.

Limit setting   Setting out, in a non-punitive way, what is and is not acceptable in another's behaviour, and informing of the consequences of transgression. Ideally, the nurse and the patient should agree on the limit setting programme.

Mental Health Act (1983)   The law as it relates to the care and treatment of patients suffering from mental disorder, which includes mental illness, personality disorder and mental handicap.

Mental illness   A general term referring to psychotic and neurotic behaviour. The term 'psychiatric illness' is used interchangeably with this.

Mental mechanism   A psychological device to protect the being (ego) from conscious awareness of unacceptable instinctual impulses (id) and to maintain harmony with conscience (superego) and external reality.

Non-verbal communication   Any signal or behaviour that transmits a message other than by words. Non-verbal behaviour includes intonation and accent as well as such behaviours as gestures, postures and touch. Non-verbal communication can act as a substitute for speech or can enhance or contradict the spoken word.

Nurse   Someone who looks after patients in a professional context and who has had, or is still in, training for the relevant nursing specialty.

Paranoid   Refers to a patient whose thinking is characterised by suspiciousness and feelings of importance. In severe paranoia, the person may become aggressive, believing that others are trying to harm him or her.

Parent   One of the three ego states in transactional analysis. The parent ego state has two forms: the controlling parent and the nurturing parent.

Passive   Referring to behaviour characterised by inactivity or reluctance to stand up for one's rights.

Patient   In this text, the term is used to refer to any person receiving professional help in the health-care setting. Increasingly, other terms are used, such as 'client', 'resident' and 'inmate'.

Personality   The relatively enduring emotional, attitudinal and behavioural characteristics that distinguish one person from another.

Precipitating factors   Those events external to the individual which can bring about an aggressive response.

Predisposing factors   Refers to processes which may explain a person's inclination to be aggressive in the absence of external events.

Restraint   Involves containing or limiting another person's freedom by mechanical, verbal or chemical means.

Seclusion   The confinement of a patient alone in a lockable room under supervision. It is reserved for the protection of others and/ or the patient.

Self-awareness   Being aware of one's own thoughts, feelings and behaviour. It includes an awareness of how one is seen by others and is an attribute of mental health.

Self-defence   To take reasonable measures to prevent another causing one harm or to take action to avoid or escape from an aggressor. Self-defence can also be carried out on behalf of someone else.

Self-reflection   The ability to self-monitor one's internal thoughts and feelings and external behaviour with respect to others.

Talking over   The use of verbal interventions to calm an aggressive encounter. It is an alternative to meeting force with force.

Threat   Suggesting by word and/or deed that something unpleasant is about to or could happen to another.

Threatening A menacing appearance or manner or, indeed, any circumstance that constitutes a threat to another.

Time out Refers to time away from reinforcement. This is designed to reduce the likelihood of current behaviour continuing and to reduce the probability of that behaviour returning.

Transactional analysis A way of studying personality and interaction in humans. It is also a method of treatment. Eric Berne, in the 1950s, was its originator.

Violence This term refers to purely physical acts of aggression.

1
The Concept of Aggression

Key Points

- Aggression is normally regarded in negative terms. It is a description of behaviour. We must strive for objectivity in describing another person as aggressive.

- Assertion is a possible strategy in responding to aggression.

- Aggression and fear may be provoked, depending on the magnitude of the threatening situation.

- Anger is the feeling component of aggressive behaviour. While growing up, people are taught to suppress anger, but failure to acknowledge feelings may result in loss of control of one's emotions.

- Expression of anger does not have to be destructive or at the expense of others. More acceptable alternatives can be learned.

- Behaviour is learned in a socio-interpersonal context. People are as much a product of the social environment as of their biology.

AGGRESSION AS NEGATIVE BEHAVIOUR

Aggression is a difficult concept to define. The term's scientific usage, let alone its popular meaning, is unclear. Some authorities take aggression to mean physical attack on another or behaviour directed towards and causing physical injury to another. The collective wisdom of Klama (1988) is salutary here as he cautions:

> The closer we get to humans, the more difficult it becomes to do justice to the complexity of the behavioural interactions that may be involved in aggression.

The definition of aggressive behaviour used throughout this book is that of the infliction of harm, or threat of harm or injury, either physical or psychological, upon another. The definition encompasses, firstly, physical aggression, also known as assault, battery or violence and, secondly, passive aggression such as sarcasm and racism. It is also intended to refer to inwardly directed aggression, such as in suicide and deliberate self-harm. These latter topics are not addressed at length in this text; instead we concentrate on nursing responses to outwardly expressed aggression.

We have opted for a definition of aggression that is in keeping with nursing's use of the term. In nursing, aggressive behaviour invariably has negative connotations, but it is worth considering everyday events that we should, perhaps, not view so negatively. The person pushing through to the front of a crowd may be seen as aggressive or simply standing up for his or her rights. Here, the way one describes someone else's behaviour may depend upon the viewpoint adopted. This difficulty in interpreting acts is also illustrated in politics: an aggressor may be viewed as a hero or a terrorist depending on which side of the political fence one stands. Whenever nurses describe a person's behaviour as aggressive, it is vital that they are mindful of the subjective influences affecting them. The implicit aversion to aggression as negative behaviour also means that at the times when society condones aggression, it is not described as such. Polite substitutes are preferred, so that terms like 'police control' or 'police tactics' are used rather than 'police aggression'. Similarly, nurses talk of 'intervention', 'restraint' and 'setting boundaries' to describe their aggressive behaviour.

However, there are a few occasions when aggression is seen in a positive light. For example, we may admire people's aggressive defence of their principles or a mother's aggression to protect her offspring from danger. In sport, a commentator admiringly remarked on a cricketer's performance:

Alan Lamb was aggressive when he went after that one.

Here, aggression is associated with its function in defending something seen as worth preserving – a right, a principle, another human being or the pursuit of excellence in sport. Aggression can also have a neutral meaning, as in 'an aggressive early morning run'.

The above considerations are important when one is judging another's behaviour. How we decide that another person is aggressive sometimes depends more on our own viewpoint than on the characteristics of the act itself. Awareness of this will help us to monitor the quality of our judgements and enable nursing staff to adopt the most therapeutic approach.

AGGRESSION AND ASSERTION

Unfortunately, the words aggression and assertion are used synonymously by some people. Of course, assertion refers to the ability to express one's views in a clear, confident, direct manner, without denying the rights of others. By implication, an aggressive manner fails to acknowledge the other's rights, and a passive response fails to acknowledge one's own rights. Assertive behaviour can mean trying to resolve problems without using manipulation or threats, and it can mean handling criticisms and uncertainty calmly. Furthermore, assertion can help us to refuse requests without feeling guilty or to ask for help when it is needed without feeling inadequate.

Being assertive is usually preferable to being either aggressive or passive. Passivity, in a member of staff for example, may well serve to reinforce a belief that one is prepared to disregard oneself for the sake of another. In patients, it could be said that passive responses are just as undesirable as aggression as they can cause resentment and even lead to an 'explosive' outburst later.

The subject of assertion is raised here for two reasons. Firstly, understanding assertion helps to show that aggressive behaviour ought not to be tolerated, especially as a long-term strategy for dealing with others. Secondly, assertion may be used in response to aggression in certain situations. However, it is important to appreciate that the interpretation of behaviours depends *as much* on a value judgement by the interpreter as on the nature of the behaviour. The dangers of making value judgements applies to both aggressive and assertive behaviours, and advanced skills are needed to prevent an intended assertive behaviour from sounding condescending or patronising. Some behaviours are easy to identify as either assertive, aggressive or passive. Table 1 shows some examples of each behaviour as provoked by the same stimulus.

One must remember that the examples in Table 1 are suggested for particular contexts. Our actions usually have a non-verbal component which we cannot convey here. Instead, the intention is largely to introduce a sense of the scope for using assertion in managing aggression, which might prompt further study. Learning to be assertive is not easy, and requires practice and

Table 1 Types of response

Aggressive	Passive	Assertive
Non-verbal indicators		
Points	Fidgets	Arms and hands relaxed by side
Stares/glares	Looks away or down	Level eye contact
Stiff upright posture	Slumped posture	Confident, upright appearance
Loud voice	Quiet, whining voice	Clear and calm speech of medium tone
Rapid speech	Hesitant speech	Even tone of voice; spaced comments
Verbal indicators		
'Look *you*'	'Excuse me . . . sorry . . .'	'I believe . . .'
'Do it *this* way'	'I wonder . . . do you mind?'	'I'd like us to look at the issues'
'Go *on*, say your piece'	Silence	'I'd like to hear your views'
Swearing	Uses words designed to please or not cause a fuss	Can keep frustrations under control

continuous commitment. We would not wish to imply that assertiveness is always a viable option – sometimes it will escalate the encounter rather than manage it – and, of course, it is unusual for someone to be assertive in every situation. However, in the context of aggression, the skilled carer needs to be able to choose from a range of options.

FIGHT AND FLIGHT RESPONSE

Reactions to threats are not automatically met by aggression. Fleeing, because of fear, could be the preferred response. In animal studies, it has been suggested that being afraid and being aggressive may, instead of being seen as two separate responses, be variants of a single response (Archer, 1967 in Swanson, 1976). Which response occurs will depend on the extent of the discrepancy between what the animal found and what it expected to find. In humans, similar explanations can account for some aggressive behaviour. Informing a patient on the day of his proposed discharge that he has to stay for another day because of transport difficulties may result in a hostile response. However, a patient who has to stay in hospital for at least another week for further investigations is likely to have a fear response only when the possible implications of a longer stay are realised. Being prepared beforehand may have reduced the discrepancy between, on the one hand, the expectation of discharge and, on the other, the reality of a longer hospital stay. Being frustrated in attaining a goal can also be considered as a discrepancy between what is expected (a reward) and what is obtained (i.e. no reward) (Swanson, 1976). Further support for the nearness of fear and aggression is seen when one considers the common experience of being both angry and afraid at the same time.

AGGRESSION AND EMOTION

Aggression can be seen as a manifestation of an underlying emotional state called anger. People commonly have feelings of anger, in the same way as they have any other emotional experience – love, sadness, joy, etc. When emotional, physiological and psychological changes are experienced, one might feel aroused, with accompanying physical changes such as increased heart rate, dry mouth, muscle tension or tremor.

Often, it is not enough simply to feel an emotion; there is also an urge to express it. In the case of love, this can be seen in the desire to kiss the loved 'object'. When angry, someone may hit out. As a young human being matures, he or she is taught to control emotions and that there is a correct time and place for their expression. Even the intensity of the emotion itself is regulated; it is acceptable to cry at a funeral but uninhibited wailing would be frowned upon, at least in many Western cultures.

Thus, the message generally conveyed is that anger is a negative emotion, to be suppressed. Yet it could be argued that the denial and suppression of 'negative' feelings is a recipe for disaster as it means losing control of the emotions and leads to behaviour the reasons for which one may not always be consciously aware of. Aggression may be displaced onto innocent others, or one might act in ways to relieve tension (for example heavy drinking) that have damaging long-term consequences. It seems best that people learn to acknowledge their feelings, regardless of whether they are good or bad; only then will it be possible to act on them in a rational way. Inward acknowledgement of angry feelings (or other emotions) is the first step. A commitment to self-awareness, slow and painful though that may be, is the best chance that there is of loading the die in favour of rationality and choice in our actions.

THE NEED TO EXPRESS AGGRESSION

It can be stated with complete confidence that the potential for aggression is present in everyone and that few people are entirely free of angry thoughts and feelings. Most have become aggressive at some time in response to another's threat, to relieve tension and frustration, in pursuance of some goal or simply to get attention. In fact, aggression is a 'natural' attribute. However, it must be stressed that the idea that aggression must be released at intervals is no longer considered relevant. What is important is the way people learn to handle aggression, both their own and that of others. It must be recognised that it is possible to win arguments and impositions without recourse to aggression – negotiation and compromise are just as effective as fighting and swearing. To lose without feeling humiliated or to bear a grudge and seek vengeance later are choices that must be made rationally. To say that human beings are 'naturally' aggressive and leave it at that ignores the contribution of the social environment in shaping and guiding people's responses. If there is such a thing as a gene for aggression, it does not follow that we cannot influence its consequences for our behaviour (Klama, 1988).

SOCIO-INTERPERSONAL ASPECTS OF AGGRESSION

It is in the social environment that collections of genes are turned into people. It was stated above in the discussion on emotions that people are taught how to respond to them; the analysis of social influence is taken a little further here. The influence of past role models can be very powerful in the way one currently behaves. Many of one's social graces tend to reflect one's family background, implying that aggressive behaviour can be 'picked up' just as readily as any other behaviour. Aggressive adults will be imitated by children observing such behaviour (Bandura, 1973). If a child learns that it is legitimate to be aggressive for whatever reason, he or she may come to rely on its use to the exclusion of alternative responses. The more success, in terms of social approval, that can be gained from being aggressive, the more likely such behaviour will be to occur. Fortunately, for most people many of the role models also display alternatives to aggression. Another powerful mitigating factor in the production of aggressive behaviour stems from the fact that most people, it would seem, like to be liked; enhancement of self-esteem is a major force for establishing relationships (DeVito, 1989). Where someone wants to be valued by another person, he or she will behave in ways likely to secure the other person's favourable impressions. Aggression normally elicits negative signals from others, consequently reducing its likelihood. This is particularly true when we are among people whom we value. In such situations we are being rewarded for not being aggressive. We obtain social approval by being pleasant, listening to what the other says, showing concern, etc. – all behaviours that are incompatible with being aggressive. In general terms, it could be said that any activity that is 'rewarding' is likely to be repeated.

To illustrate further the effects of the social environment on aggression, Schachter and Singer (1962) investigated the relationship between physiological arousal and psychological feeling. These researchers suggested that subjects interpreted their arousal with respect to the prevailing socio-psychological climate and that arousal on its own was not enough to specify the emotion felt. In this experiment, subjects were told they were testing a new vitamin but were, in fact, given either a harmless placebo or adrenalin, which was intended to put them in a state of physiological arousal. Subjects were then divided into different test groups and exposed to 'happy' and 'angry' social settings. Results indicated that subjects' responses reflected the mood of the setting they were in. The effect of the adrenalin was only to enhance the subjects' response, not to 'inform' them whether they were happy or angry.

From these results, it would appear that feelings of arousal are dependent for their interpretation on the mood of the setting in which they arise. However, the more usual scenarios in aggressive encounters are of subjects becoming aroused in response to a stimulus of some sort, and subsequent responses are dependent on a whole range of possible socio-interpersonal factors. For instance, you may believe that throwing litter is wrong. Along comes someone who drops a crisp packet on the ground; this 'makes' you angry. Deciding your next move may be problematic. It is likely to depend on many considerations, such as the size and appearance of the offender – might they retaliate if you ask them to bin the litter? Or it may depend on your success in the past in stopping people leaving litter. Consider, now, the same situation where the perpetrator of the offence is your new boss. Might this information alter the response? We could go on thinking about socio-interpersonal mediating factors such as skills in challenging another, wanting to impress an audience, etc. Even when patients are ill, with low tolerance levels, it is as much the attention at the socio-interpersonal level that determines the outcome of the interaction as a concern simply for physical or psychological factors. It would appear that we are more a product of our environment than we perhaps care to admit.

AGGRESSION AND THE THREAT TO SELF

For many of us, the aggression we encounter from others is, more often than not, far from life-threatening. Rather, it is a threat only at the intrapersonal level. When we are told off or spoken to harshly, we react to protect our 'good name'. It would appear that saving face is now just as important as saving life. The old adage 'Sticks and stones may break my bones but names will never hurt me' seems, therefore, not to be true, although our politicians appear to illustrate it well. Some of the most vitriolic abuse is seen in politics, yet outside the political arena the same people can be seen on friendly terms, so it might be argued that the roles we assume exert very powerful forces on our behaviour. Many of us, however, are not so resilient, and even 'minor' slights can have lasting effects.

There are two messages here. Firstly, we need to be able to protect ourselves at the intrapersonal level when aggression does arise. Secondly, we need interpersonal skills to help the other not to suffer loss of face when an alternative, non-aggressive course of action is sought. In situations where physical attack happens or is likely, of course, one requires an awareness of how to protect oneself by physical means (i.e. restraint or escape), yet even in these situations attentions to inner thoughts and feelings will provide the calmness required to effect resolutions.

Further Reading

The first two books in the following list together provide a comprehensive account of past and present thought on the nature of aggression. The older text emphasises the instinctual nature of aggression in many aspects of our behaviour, while the Klama text takes an optimistic view of the potential for humans to live cooperatively.

Klama J (1988) *Aggression: Conflict in Animals and Humans Reconsidered*. Essex: Longman Scientific and Technical.

Storr A (1968) *Human Aggression*. Harmondsworth: Penguin Books.

Bond M (1987) Being Assertive (Workbook and Reader); Unit 18 in *Managing Care*. London: Distance Learning Centre, South Bank Polytechnic.

Lindenfield G (1986) *Assert Yourself*. Ilkley: Self-Help Associates. (A concise introduction to assertiveness and assertiveness training. It includes various exercises and activities. Information on courses in assertiveness can be obtained from Health Education Units, public libraries or MIND, 22 Harley Street, London, W1N 2ED.)

Rakos R (1990) *Assertive Behaviour: Theory, Research and Training*. London: Routledge. (A well-referenced manual for those looking beyond the 'pop' psychology status that assertiveness training enoys in some quarters.)

Tutt, N (ed.) (1976) *Violence*. London: Department of Health, HMSO. (A good and varied selection of essays on issues related to the topic of violence.)

Part I

REFLECT

An important part of staff preparation for dealing with aggression involves raising their awareness of the roles of the self, the other party and the environment in bringing about aggression. 'The other party' here refers to the aggressor; what he or she brings to the encounter can be thought of as the *predisposing* factors in the aggressive incident. 'The environment' includes everything in the aggressor's surroundings: other patients, visitors and staff as well as the physical features generally taken to make up the environment for all of us. These may be seen as the *precipitating* factors. Gaining a qualitative understanding of these factors and the interplay between them is the first stage of the management process. The keyword is REFLECT, i.e. be prepared to acknowledge the various complex factors influencing aggressive responses.

2
Self-awareness

Key Points

- Recognising how we may contribute to another person's aggression is the first step in aggression management training.

- Self-awareness arises through self-reflection and feedback from others.

- Interactions can be understood in terms of transactional analysis.

- Staff in demanding environments should evaluate their need for help to reduce stress, and decide how this can be done.

- Stress reduction techniques should acknowledge the intellectual, emotional and physical aspects of the self.

Self-awareness, in simple terms, refers to the knowledge we have of ourselves. It is vital that a nurse understands how his or her behaviour is perceived by other people. Aggression rarely occurs in a vacuum, away from the influence of others, and staff should engage in continuous self-reflection to enable them to monitor their behaviour. Those who regularly monitor their behaviour have been shown to be effective in a range of social situations (Dickson, Hargie and Horrow, 1989). Far from indulging in introversion, the so-called reflective practitioner uses his or her experience to improve future effectiveness (Schon, 1983). Self-reflection should be a lifelong endeavour, and nurses must develop this skill if they are to offer a therapeutic service to patients.

Anyone can become aggressive when feeling provoked or threatened. Often it is not clear just who is being aggressive: a patient's self-assertion can be mislabelled as 'aggressive' by nurses who see their authority challenged.

Try this exercise.

ACTIVITY 1

The behaviour of others can be an important factor in aggressive encounters. Spend a few minutes listing some of the things that you could say and do to make another person aggressive. Then list what other people could say and do to make you aggressive. Now see the discussion below.

Discussion
Here are the responses made by a group of student nurses when asked, 'What do others do to make you angry?':

Turn up late for appointments.
Ignore me.
Talk about themselves when I want to talk about myself.
Waste resources, like gas, electricity or water.
Pick their nose.
Squeeze toothpaste unevenly.
Produce shoddy workmanship.
Be over-fussy.
Be indecisive.
Nag.
Auntie refusing to put the heating on.
People who act as if they know everything.
Telling, rather than asking me what should be done.

Given a larger sample, no doubt this list would be greatly extended. What upsets people varies, and people also vary in what they find upsetting at a given moment; for example, I might welcome a little horseplay down at the pub, but find it irksome when I am ill.

This exercise has been designed to focus attention on the things that others could do to upset you and to increase your awareness of how your behaviour might upset others. It is important to think carefully about your behaviour as, firstly, it may provoke others to become aggressive and, secondly, the way you respond to a 'provocation' will be crucial in determining the outcome. Being offhand with someone who is trying to get your attention may serve only to increase their feeling of frustration

To increase your awareness further, the following exercise is suggested.

ACTIVITY 2

Ask a close friend to write down, firstly, the things that he or she likes about your behaviour and, secondly, the things he or she finds irritating. Compare these to a list of your own perceptions of your behaviour. Ideally, this sort of exercise should be carried out in a facilitated group over a long period, with a leader skilled in group dynamics. Nevertheless, it can heighten awareness in some small measure. Now see the discussion below.

Discussion
Asking for both positive and negative comments makes it more likely that people will say what they really think, as there is opportunity to achieve a balance between positive and negative statements. A possible problem with these and similar exercises is that you may find out things you do not wish to hear. Thus, some nurses may find such exercises threatening, as they fear being evaluated and find it difficult to cope with negative feedback. However, unless we reflect on our own behaviour, we will continue to *react*, rather than thinking first and then acting. Below are some suggestions for giving and receiving feedback. Bear these in mind when thinking about the above exercise.

Giving effective feedback:
- Say something positive to begin and end with.
- Comment on the actual behaviour observed. Talk about the things you saw and heard, not what you imagined or inferred, thus avoiding interpretations. Think in terms of rejecting the behaviour rather than the person.
- Avoid vague general statements. 'This was awful' does nothing to indicate to the individual why you have come to those conclusions.
- Make it relevant. Comment on things that the person might be able to change. Telling someone that you do not like the way he smiles is less than constructive.
- Choose a time and place to give feedback when the recipient is most likely to be able to make the best use of it.
- Don't advise or judge.
- Use feedback sparingly. Criticism can hurt, even if it is constructive.
- Don't forget that feedback also says something about the person giving it.

Receiving feedback:
- Listen to the comments.
- Avoid defensiveness. Do not make excuses.
- Ask for clarification.

- Get a balanced view. See if other people think the same way.
- Ask for other feedback if it does not seem forthcoming.
- Decide what use you can make of the comments. You could try to modify certain aspects of your behaviour, such as improving your listening skills.
- Consider how important the comments are to you. Where professional practice is not an issue, there are individual freedoms; maybe you will choose to continue to wave your arm around when you speak, even though it upsets a particular listener.
- Thank the giver of the feedback. This gives approval to the general principle of feedback, which is an invaluable practice in any context where relationships are important.

Stuart and Sundeen (1983) suggest that a lack of self-awareness can result in nurses making non-therapeutic responses when faced with threatening situations. They outline three main types of non-therapeutic responses: defensiveness, 'pulling rank'/condescension and avoidance. Read the two cameos below and make a note for each of the type of non-therapeutic response before reading the discussion that follows.

1. Mr Webb, on learning that he has to stay in hospital for longer than at first thought, complains to the nurse about 'this latest inconvenience'. The nurse tries to reassure him by explaining, 'We are only trying to ensure that when you are discharged you will be as fit as possible'. 'But they should have told me in the beginning they weren't certain how long I'd be here. Now I don't know when I'm going to get back to work', retorts the patient, by now obviously upset and angry. The nurse tries to explain why it is difficult to be sure how long a particular patient's stay will last, and goes on to say, 'Our concern, Mr Webb, is to do the best job possible'. Mr Webb goes silent.

2. Mrs Thomas, a well-to-do lady in her early forties, repeatedly requests, 'Have a look at my dressing, nurse. I think it needs changing'. Eventually, a nurse looks at Mrs Thomas' dressing and finds that it does, in fact, need changing. Mrs Thomas reacts angrily when the nurse arrives to change her dressing. 'It seems you have to decide for yourself when things need attention around here. Not only that, you have to plead with a nurse to get anything done'. The nurse immediately comments, 'There was no need to change your dressing immediately as your wound is healing as well as can be expected. In a busy ward like this we have to prioritise so that everyone is given the best care for their particular needs'.

Discussion

The first scenario exemplifies defensiveness. Stuart and Sundeen comment on such behaviour thus: 'The nurse interprets the patient's anger as a personal attack and immediately tries to explain her action to prove that the perceived attack is unjustified'. The patient was probably worried about his health and wondering if he was ever going to be discharged. That, combined with the fact that his hopes for discharge are now dashed, may have led to his hostile reaction. It is unlikely that his outburst was intended for that particular nurse; it is more probable that she just happened to be the most convenient person available to vent his frustration on.

In the second scenario, the nurse's response can be seen as 'pulling rank'. The nurse sees herself as the one with authority in the health care setting. The nurse responds, as in the first scenario, only to the superficial meaning of the situation and does not attempt to respond to the patient's underlying thoughts and feelings. Mrs Thomas probably feels resentful at what she sees as neglectful behaviour on the part of the nurses, and may also be feeling anxious and vulnerable. Likewise, the nurse's behaviour may be seen as condescending as she assumes an air of superiority. Belittling is another example of condescension and might be seen in the case of an uncooperative adult patient who is reprimanded as if he or she were a child. In so doing, the nurse discounts the patient's feelings altogether.

Pulling rank may also be seen in nurses who adopt a 'macho' attitude towards aggression. This results in attempts to over-control the patient, and to feelings that the nurse can cope with any encounter. Staff with this attitude often 'have a problem with their own aggression' and adopt a confrontational approach to patients, which can spark off aggression.

In avoidance behaviour, the nurse may draw on several devices to avoid recognising the patient's anger. For example, the nurse may try to avoid any contact with the patient, and in situations where interaction is inevitable, the nurse will change the subject as soon as any hint of patient anger is perceived. Stuart and Sundeen (1983) neatly illustrate avoidance behaviour in the following passage:

> The patient said to the nurse as she changed his dressing, 'You know, I think my doctor is botching my case. This infection is no better. I think he's a real quack'. The nurse continues with the procedure and after a moment said, 'Did your wife visit yesterday, Mr A? She seems such a nice person – so concerned about you'. Mr A sighed and

closed his eyes as the nurse completed the procedure. Later the nurse said to a friend, 'That Mr A is a strange one. He hardly responds at all when you try and talk to him'.

Travelbee (1976) suggests that patients become angry when nurses neglect to see them as individuals. Patients can be categorised by a process of human reduction. For example, they may be perceived as illnesses – 'Have you done the obs on the chole in room 3?' – or as tasks – 'I have to do the dressing in room 1'. Attitudes such as these are inadvertently transmitted to the patient. We can all recall incidents where we, too, may have portrayed the above attitudes by our mechanical approach during patient admission: 'Name, address, type of accommodation, past medical history . . .'. This information could be elicited in a far more therapeutic way. As well as putting the patient at ease, careful attention to the interview process will enable the nurse to appreciate the special needs of each patient. In a study reported by Lucas and Folstein (1980) on 100 medical in-patients, it was found that 49% scored positively for emotional distress. Nurses questioned about these patients failed to recognise 41% of cases.

Lyttle (1986) cites two extreme examples of staff who may fail to acknowledge patients as individuals: Nurses Saccharine and Vinegar. Nurse Saccharine is characterised as being motherly in a superficial way, avoiding getting close to patients and exuding superficial concern. Patients are called 'pets', 'poor dears', 'darlings' or 'poor old souls'. Though well-meaning, her stock of unhelpful platitudes ('Never mind, things will look better in the morning', 'Every cloud has a silver lining') only serves to alienate patients, making them feel rejected and demeaned. Nurse Vinegar is characterised as authoritarian, rigid, emotionally inhibited and very much the 'critical parent'. This nurse expects patients and others to conform to his or her standards, has a knack of upsetting patients and is rigidly 'efficient' and task-orientated in caring for patients. Nurse Vinegar's outward rigidness masks a vulnerable personality that is easily hurt, so he or she avoids situations that might be emotionally threatening.

Of course, these two caricatures are examples of extremes, rarely seen in reality. But, as Lyttle suggests, elements of them may exist in any of us and will create barriers to effective nurse–patient relationships. Both treat the patient as a child rather than an adult, and because both encourage nurse–patient involvement at only a superficial level, they will be unable to understand patients as individuals.

Further means of understanding what might be happening in nurse–patient interactions is provided by transactional analysis

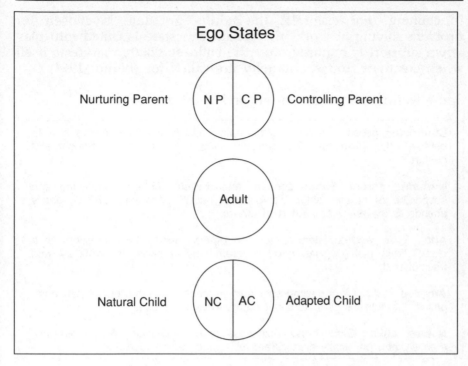

Fig 2.1 The structure of the personality

(TA), which is seen as a method of analysing social intercourse. Very briefly, TA suggests that we each have three ego states, i.e. states of mind. These are termed 'parent ego state', 'adult ego state' and 'child ego state', and each involves recognisable sets of related attitudes and behaviours (Figure 2.1). The parent ego state may be seen in one of two forms: the controlling parent is critical and has a set of rigid rules that restrict the activity of others, whereas the nurturing parent manifests sympathy, support, caring and concern for self and others. The adult ego state is characterised as being autonomous, adaptable and intelligent. A person in this state can evaluate incoming data objectively and respond to events calmly and thoughtfully. The child ego state has two forms. The adapted child conforms to the demands and impositions of others; this is seen in such behaviours as sulking, withdrawal and alternating aggressive and rebellious behaviours. The natural child, on the other hand, is spontaneous and acts freely without regard for the consequences. Ego states can be seen as coherent behaviour displays, i.e. the ego state currently in operation is recognisable. An ability to shift from one ego state to another in response to changing circumstances signals healthy functioning. For example, the adult ego state is chosen for problem solving at work, the parent ego state is called into play when support is required, and the child ego state manifests itself when creativity and spontaneity are called for (Berne, 1964).

Some features of parent, adult and child ego states:

Controlling parent: Critical, argumentative and pushy. Tells others how to behave – 'Do it like this', 'That's a silly thing to do'. Adopts an upright, stiff posture.

Nurturing parent: Shows concern and warmth. Always welcoming and supportive of others. Asks, 'How can I help?', 'Are you OK?'. Readily attends to the physical comfort of others.

Adult: Calm and confident. Listens to others' views. Asks questions in a clear, direct fashion. Has good problem solving skills. Is confident and unemotional.

Adapted child: Shows withdrawn and/or rebellious behaviour. Often complains. Expects things to turn out badly. Tries to please.

Natural child: Often noisy, excitable and uninhibited. Wants to play; mentally and physically alert. Creative. Laughs and chuckles.

Some individuals can get 'stuck' in one ego state, tending to use the same, favourite behaviours in most situations. The constant parent is an example. Other individuals may have two or more ego states operating at once, often below the level of awareness. The adult may believe that the fantasies, wishes and impulsive behaviour of the child are part of the adult state. If a person loses control of his or her ego states, the ability for autonomy and self-determination is lost.

Your own personality can be illustrated by use of an egogram (Figure 2.2 after Dusay, 1977).

Figures 2.3 and 2.4 give space for you to map out your own egogram at work and at home. It is not unusual to have a different personality profile at work from that at home, which is to be expected as the two situations can call for different sets of roles. However, whether at work or at home, the important consideration is the nature of transactions with others.

One of the purposes of interactions, or transactions, is social contact and approval. We all have both a biological and psychological need for recognition. Berne introduced to TA the term 'stroking', by which he referred to an act that implied recognition of another's presence. Stroking may be verbal, as in a greeting,

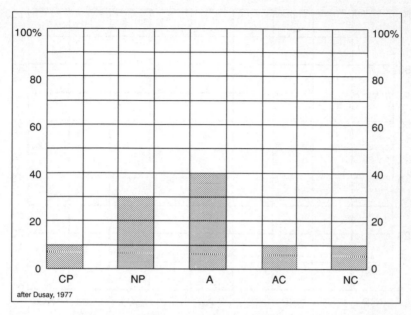

Fig 2.2 An example of an egogram; each ego state is shown as a percentage of a typical day's total interactions

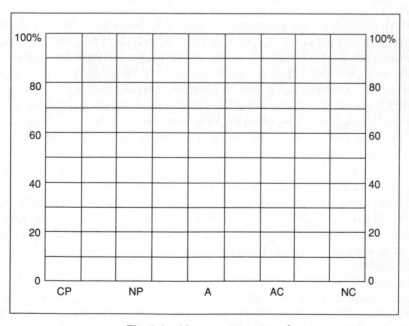

Fig 2.3 My egogram at work

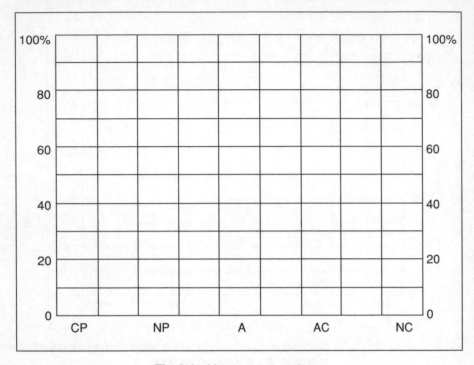

Fig 2.4 My egogram at home

or non-verbal, as in gestures or other behaviours. An exchange of strokes constitutes a transaction, which is the unit of social intercourse. In securing strokes, we engage in various activities, from well-defined rituals, such as when two people greet one another in passing, to more elaborate transactions (psychological games) where there are ulterior motives and hidden pay-offs.

We all need strokes, ideally positive ones, where a 'You're an OK person' message is delivered. However, if positive strokes are not forthcoming, negative strokes are preferable to no strokes at all. Some people can get 'locked' into receiving predominantly negative strokes; they constantly end up as a 'victim' and perpetuate their life pattern by eliciting negative strokes from others (Lange, 1978). Steiner (1970) describes positive strokes as 'warm fuzzies' and negative strokes as 'cold pricklies', as these are convenient ways to imagine the emotional overtones that go with each.

As noted above, an exchange of strokes constitutes a transaction, which is the unit of social intercourse (Berne, 1964). Transactions take place between ego states. TA determines the ways in which an ego state in one person communicates with the

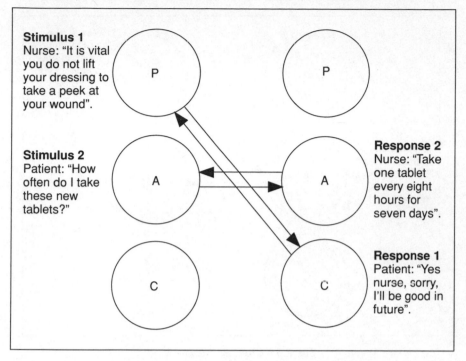

Stimulus 1
Nurse: "It is vital you do not lift your dressing to take a peek at your wound".

Stimulus 2
Patient: "How often do I take these new tablets?"

Response 2
Nurse: "Take one tablet every eight hours for seven days".

Response 1
Patient: "Yes nurse, sorry, I'll be good in future".

Fig 2.5 Complementary transactions

ego state in another person. There are usually three main types of transaction: complementary, crossed and ulterior. A complementary transaction is one in which the initiator of the stimulus receives a response from the ego state which has been addressed. Examples of complementary transactions are given in Figure 2.5. In fact, there are nine possible types of complementary transactions; PP, PA, PC, AP, AA, AC, CP, CA and CC.

In crossed transactions (Figure 2.6) the response comes from a different ego state from the one originally addressed, or the response is directed to a different ego state from the one which initiated the communication. In theory at least, complementary transactions can go on indefinitely, whereas in crossed transactions communication is usually broken off. One or both parties may feel misunderstood or, indeed, angry.

Ulterior transactions (Figure 2.7) hide the real motives for the transaction. The social interaction may appear ordinary, but covertly there is a hidden agenda, which will have a negative pay-off for one or both parties.

Note that transactions can occur without words being spoken: a gesture or 'manner' can communicate very powerfully.

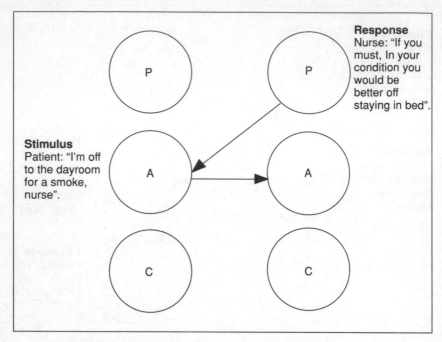

Fig 2.6 Crossed transactions

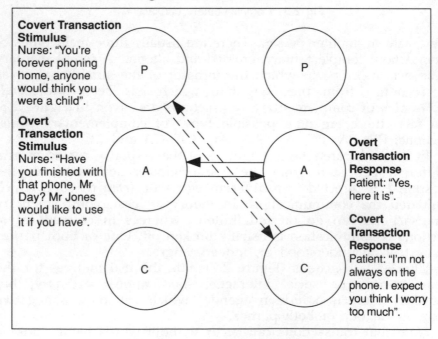

Fig 2.7 An ulterior transaction

Transactional analysis can have relevance for nursing in the context of aggression in a number of ways, four of which are briefly discussed here. First, knowledge and understanding of how we present ourselves to patients in terms of our unique parent, adult and child profile will give us the insight necessary to effect the changes that might be required in our nurse–patient interactions. The nurse–patient relationship calls for many complementary interactions. When patients are very ill, it may be appropriate to relate to patients in the role of the nurturing parent, but as the patient becomes less dependent, adult type transactions will be more therapeutic. Excessively maternalistic or paternalistic environments are likely to produce conflicts when patients seek autonomy.

Secondly, we can think of what our needs are with respect to receiving strokes. Are there some types of stroke we seek regardless of cost? Do we need frequent strokes from our patients, perhaps in the form of expressed gratitude? What happens when these are not forthcoming – do we engineer encounters so that patients have little option but to say 'Thanks'?

Thirdly, patients, too, will have a need for strokes. Patients who are left alone sometimes become demanding and abusive in an attempt to elicit attention (a stroke in the terms of TA). In such situations, any response from the nurse may be interpreted by the patient as a stroke. It is important that patients receive attention when they are not demanding because there is a tendency for strokes to reinforce whatever behaviours brought them about. This means that if we give attention only when someone is behaving 'badly', this behaviour may be seen as necessary to gain attention. Taking time out to talk with patients and showing concern for their comfort needs are two ways in which nurses can give patients 'warm fuzzies'.

Fourthly, caring for patients who are unable and/or unwilling to give nurses strokes can place great strain on the nurse–patient relationship. Lange (1978) suggests that staff members become unhappy and disgruntled when a patient seems unappreciative – 'You can't do anything to please her', 'She never says "Thanks"', 'He won't let you help him'. When feelings like these predominate, staff generally withdraw from the unrewarding patient, leaving that individual with his or her own (often lifelong) pattern of unsatisfactory interpersonal relationships. Lange points out the need for periodic evaluation and super-vision, as well as acknowledgement by co-workers, in meeting the nurse's need for recognition in demanding and difficult conditions. Morale is maintained when staff receive positive strokes in the form of recognition of their worth and appreciation of their hard work.

Nurses' ability to recognise patients' needs may be compromised, too, when they are in a hurry. Being too busy may result in failure to notice people's concerns: for example providing enough information of the right type in good time may prevent anger building up. Patients can be helped to cope with the frustrations of a long wait by explaining the reasons for the delays and by asking them if there is anything that could make their wait as comfortable as possible. If patients are left without information, they will interpret the situation as they see it: some will think they have been forgotten while others may feel incensed. Volicer and Bohannon (1974) emphasise the need for good nurse–patient communication. They comment that staff can directly affect patients' perceptions of stressful hospital experiences. In their research, patients rated 'not being told what your diagnosis is', 'not having your questions answered by staff', 'having nurses or doctors talk too fast or use words you cannot understand' and 'having the staff in too much of a hurry' among the most stressful events. The implication here is that greater attention to communication with patients can lessen their anxiety. This point is well illustrated in one study where a simple programme of counselling provided by coronary care nurses significantly reduced anxiety and depression in male first myocardial infarction patients and reduced anxiety in their partners (Thompson, 1989).

No discussion of self-awareness would be complete without devoting some space to the subject of attitudes. The attitudes we hold towards others can be seen as reflecting the feelings we have for them (Argyle, 1988). Anger is an emotion, while being angry with someone is an interpersonal attitude. As nurses, we have to deal with an enormous number of patients with various conditions and personalities. It is not surprising, therefore, that we respond better to some patients and their conditions than to others. The available literature on nurses' perception of illnesses would appear to bear out this view. For instance, incontinence (Stockwell, 1972), mutilation (Simpson et al, 1979; Stockwell, 1972) and mental disturbance (Simpson et al, 1979) have been linked to nurses' negative attitudes towards patients with these problems, whereas illnesses that offer a challenge to nurses' skills, and conditions that respond rapidly to treatment, are viewed positively. However, we are rarely in a position to choose whom we nurse, so if we are to treat everyone with the same degree of care and attention, it is highly probable that there will be some occasions when we have to mask our underlying negative feelings towards a patient. Unless one is a very good actor, it will be extremely difficult to hide one's true feelings for very long. Sooner or later they will 'leak' out through non-verbal channels, so that the attitude is inadvertently transmitted to the patient. This might help to account for some of the difficulties we have with some of our patients.

DeVito (1989) argues that our non-verbal behaviour is 'highly believable'. He goes on to assert that people readily believe non-verbal behaviours, even when they contradict verbal messages. Ekman et al (1976) asked student nurses to watch an unpleasant film, following which they were instructed to tell an interviewer that they had just watched a pleasant film. The students' non-verbal responses were compared to those of a control group who had reported on a pleasant film. Findings suggest that the deception group used more hand movements and shrugs and had an increased voice pitch. Although we normally get more information from facial cues, Ekman and Friesen (1969) note that, in deceptive situations when head and body cues conflict, body movements will 'leak' more than facial expressions and are a better indicator of an individual's emotional state. These 'leaky' behaviours seem to bear out what Freud said in 1905, 'If his lips are silent he chatters with his fingertips; betrayal oozes out of him at every pore'. If we want to convey friendliness and liking for another, Argyle (1988) suggests that we pay more attention to the following non-verbal behaviours:

- *Proximity*: closer, forward lean if seated.
- *Orientation*: more direct, but side by side for some situations.
- *Gaze*: more gaze and mutual gaze.
- *Facial expression*: more smiling.
- *Gestures*: head nods, lively movements.
- *Posture*: open with arms stretched towards the other as opposed to arms on hips or folded.
- *Touch*: more touch in an appropriate manner.
- *Tone of voice*: higher pitch, upward pitch contour, pure tone.

Argyle also includes self-disclosure as an important verbal component of friendliness. Of course, the above behaviours need to be attuned to the particular situation. The same behaviours can appear too friendly in some situations or too distant in others.

The way we use individual non-verbal behaviours is important too. Nurses have to learn how to touch patients in a way that is reassuring but not sexual, and how to observe but not stare. Choosing the appropriate words and learning to use non-verbal signals are two important components of the social skill of conveying positive attitudes. To improve our non-verbal performance, we can use a variety of methods, including modelling skilled performers, self-monitoring (*in vivo* and by observing ourselves on video or even in the mirror), graded practice, seeking feedback from others and involvement in social skills training groups.

Finally, another important consideration is to acknowledge to ourselves the attitudes we hold towards our patients. However, sometimes even for ourselves, these are not easy to identify, as they can be concealed by resorting to mental mechanisms. For example, we may not spend much time with a patient because his wound is offensive or because his mood is depressing. But rationalisation occurs, and instead of acknowledging this as a reason for keeping away, we account for our behaviour in terms of being too busy, or we use projection and tell ourselves that he does not like us. Meanwhile, the true reason remains in the background, probably at a subconscious level. If we see worth in all our patients, we will be motivated to interact with them in a positive sense, regardless of their particular circumstances.

Inconsistent staff behaviour encourages patients to test or check out staff attempts to adopt therapeutic approaches. This highlights the need, yet again, for clearly thought-out written care plans. Of course, they still need to be implemented consistently, but they provide the means by which this can occur. The use of care plans, however, does not lessen the need for staff with well-developed interpersonal skills. Being vague or half-heartedly following a plan leaves the patient in an uncertain position.

In putting a case for consistency we are, of course, not adovcating an inflexible approach to care. Strict, authoritarian environments could actually encourage aggression, as patients see no other way to meet their needs. In situations where a patient is aggressive, it is particularly important that staff behaviour is seen to be firm, fair and flexible. Similarly, overdramatic staff responses may actually encourage aggression. There may be a sense of the need to make a statement, and patients may feel a sense of powerfulness when able to elicit a flurry of staff activity. In some cases, it may just be that patients will imitate the 'aggressive' behaviour of staff in response to conflict. Clearly, we have to strike a balance between *laissez-faire* and authoritarian environments, both of which are anti-therapeutic in the management of aggression.

Busy, demanding work environments may also affect the ability to relate therapeutically to patients. Consider the nurse who feels under stress due to pressure of work. The need to get everything done may compromise the desire to spend more time with individual patients. Lack of staff attention may tend to bring about aggression in those who feel they need to be cared for and those who find it difficult to perceive the boundaries of some of their behaviours. As a result, some patients may feel frustrated and may 'act up' to get the attention they feel they need. Lack of staff attention may also mean that faulty behaviours go unchallenged, leading to patients feeling that anything goes. In some instances, it will certainly be realistic to ask for more staff as a way of reducing the incidence and severity of work-related stress. Alternatively, it may be worth trying to alter the structure of the working day: taking more short breaks, rearranging workload or perhaps altering shift patterns to improve staff numbers when patients most need help. Often, it helps if nurses share with others how they feel. This could be accomplished more formally through regular group meetings devoted to exploring the work situation, especially perhaps its stressful aspects (Kornfeld, 1969). Out of work, engaging in a favourite relaxation activity will help.

Walton (1984) suggests we need to manage our stress at three levels – the intellectual level, the emotional level and the physical level – and suggests stress reduction steps for each level.

The intellectual level:

1. Formulate realistic goals, the value of which you appreciate.
2. Sort out what you want to be and do.
3. Replace old ways of working passed on to you automatically with new ones that you establish for yourself.
4. Avoid unnecessary or too frequent changes.
5. Be as honest as you can about what is going on, why it is going on and your part in it.

The emotional level:

1. Allow yourself time to admit to your feelings. Do not be ashamed of them.
2. Allow yourself to feel situations.
3. Stop being a victim. Do things you want for a change.
4. Be aware of your emotional and social contacts and your need for them.

The physical level:

1. Take care of your body.
2. Improve your breathing.

3. Make sure you get enough exercise.
4. Make sure your diet is adequate and balanced.
5. Try out meditation and other relaxation techniques.

Reducing our stress will have important implications in a more general sense, too. Patients are reassured when nurses themselves convey emotional stability. It is worth emphasising that reassurance does not necessarily mean words. As Frost (1974) has said, 'Anyone can hand out advice, but it is the skilled nurse that can sit quietly and without tension while the patient struggles with his thoughts'. Sometimes our usual methods of controlling stress may not be enough, and we may need expert advice, for example assertiveness and anxiety management training. However, for some the stress inherent in the job is felt to be too great and they think about leaving. Those who experience severe distress should perhaps consider alternative areas of work if they cannot adapt. We would urge, however, that all options be carefully considered, so that the pros and cons of leaving can be weighed against those of staying in the job.

The settings in which aggression is a frequent occurrence may 'suit' some people, who are attracted to work in specialities that are seen as demanding. People with so-called type A behaviour 'prefer' environments that are challenging. Such behaviour types are said to have inappropriate ambition and to be work-orientated, competitive yet reluctant to provide self-evaluation, always in a hurry and aggressive. Those with type B behaviour show the opposite characteristics. They are relaxed and easy-going, focus on quality over quantity of work, can separate work from play and are more reflective (Reber, 1985). In aggressive environments, it is the latter characteristics we should be striving for. Unfortunately, type A people are often unaware of their behaviour. It follows that teaching the need for self-observation is a crucial first step in helping people to change. Note that environmental stress, regardless of its cause, should not be seen as something that is always present and cannot be altered. We should, as well as trying to adapt our behaviour in response to environmental demands, look at ways to reduce the environmental demands on the individual: it would be silly, for instance, to teach staff how to cope with the pressure of busy departments without also looking to see whether there were enough staff on duty to cope in the first place or to see whether other factors could be altered.

The above discussion has provided a number of examples of how our own behaviour may interfere with our attempts to provide therapeutic care. Self-monitoring should occur both during and following interactions. As you work through the remainder of this text, you will find further examples where the need for self-monitoring is emphasised.

Further Reading

Berne E (1964) *Games People Play: The Psychology of Human Relationships*. Harmondsworth: Penguin. (Provides a brief but very readable account of transactional analysis and illustrates ulterior transactions particularly well.)

Bond M (1986) *Stress and Self-Awareness: A Guide for Nurses*. London: Heinemann. (This offers a great variety of techniques and suggestions for increasing personal awareness and managing stress.)

Monet A and Lazarus R S (eds.) (1985) *Stress and Coping*. New York: Colombia University Press. (A learned text covering a wide range of topics within these fields, all suitably well-referenced.)

Rudinger E (1988) *Understanding Stress*. London: Consumers' Association. (A good general introduction. Explains the causes of stress, and includes practical help and advice on how to overcome it.)

3
Factors Precipitating Aggression

Key Points

- The behaviour of staff and other people may serve to bring about aggression.

- Aggression may be precipitated by physical factors in the patient's environment and by organisational constraints.

- Hostile responses are usually the result of many minor irritations coming together in an already vulnerable individual.

- Nurses should aim to reduce environmental triggers as far as is possible.

The idea underlying the REFLECT stage of the cycle is that greater awareness of the possible causes of aggression can lead directly to reductions in its incidence. Such reductions are possible because factors having the potential to cause aggression can sometimes be avoided or compensated for, once acknowledged. The aim of this chapter is to consider some of the causes that appear to arise outside the person, which generally include causes attributed to other people or the environment.

ACTIVITY 3

Think about a situation you have been in or a patient you have nursed. Try to recall some of the external influences that have brought about aggressive behaviour.

Now see the discussion below.

Discussion
As we saw in the above section on self-awareness, our own behaviour may trigger off patients' aggression. In fact, our

behaviour and our attitudes are very powerful socio-environmental influences on patient behaviour. But in some ways nurses do not actually have to *do* anything to affect the environment adversely. It seems simply that low staffing numbers, inexperienced staff and poor skill mix all have a bearing on the incidence and consequences of aggression. Some of the other forms of socio-environmental influence are considered in the following paragraphs.

One of the most immediate influences in the patient's environment is that of other patients. Sometimes patients may not 'get on' with one another. This may be because the behaviour brought about by a patient's illness interferes with another patient's routine, or there may simply be a personality clash. Often, the signs that all is not well are indirect. For instance, a patient may complain of sleeping badly because 'Poor Bert wasn't well again last night', or a patient may ask in an exasperated tone of voice, 'Will I be in this bay until I'm discharged?' Try and gauge patient atmosphere early to see if remedial action is required. Therapeutic interventions could involve simply moving one of the individuals to a different location. Alternatively, talking to the offended party can do much to disperse ill-feeling, as this acknowledges emotions; it could lead the way to holding an open discussion between all concerned to decide how best to resolve any differences.

Another significant influence comes from friends and relatives. They may provoke an aggressive incident amongst themselves or they may take their guilt and frustration out on staff. It can sometimes be wise to separate patients from those accompanying them, particularly when, perhaps after a drunken brawl, a patient attends an Accident and Emergency Department with a group of friends. However, the actual approach to the situation depends on the complete circumstance, and only knowledge and experience will permit the right judgement to be made. There are some situations, of course, where it would be completely inappropriate to separate patient and companion, especially where a young child is concerned.

In an existing episode of aggressive behaviour, other people, including friends, relatives and patients, may encourage the episode to be continued. Equally, they may precipitate the aggression in the first place, albeit inadvertently. The aggression may escalate because the patient wants to impress his or her audience: not losing face can be a powerful motivator to sustain hostility. Always be on the lookout for such situations and seek ways to limit the effect of the audience. Simply asking the onlookers to leave is one way of exercising some control. Further discussion of this issue is contained in the section on bystanders in Chapter 6.

A possibly less obvious influence on behaviour is over-crowding. Where many people live together, the structure should afford opportunity for any individual to be alone at times, or to have some space to call his or her own, even if only for short periods. Fried and DeFazio (1974) found that passengers on an underground train tended to favour seats that were likely to provide minimal body contact and obvious boundaries between self and other passengers. Hall (1959, in Hargie et al, 1987) suggests that, depending on the type of interaction, people have four main proximity zones, referring to the distance kept between themselves and others when interacting. These are described as: (a) the intimate zone, approximately 18 in, for people in a very close relationship; (b) the personal zone, 18 in to 4 ft, for people in a close relationship; (c) the social consultative zone, 9–12 ft, for interactions between professionals and clients; and (d) the public zone, over 12 ft, for public interactions, such as when giving a lecture. As nurses we often have to 'invade' patients' personal and intimate zones, which may cause patient distress (French, 1983). French suggests that nurses should regard an area of 2 ft around the patient's bed and bedside locker as his or her personal space and should aim to avoid invading this space as much as possible. It is useful to remember that Hall's suggestions relate to normal behaviour and that in nursing settings this is not always to be expected. Kinzel (1970) reports that prisoners convicted of violent crimes seem to require a particularly large interactive distance, and there were similar conclusions from a study involving patients suffering from schizophrenia (Horowitz et al, 1964).

Apart from direct human influences, there are many potential triggers of aggression present in the average physical setting. A lack of facilities may cause immense frustration, so waiting areas should have a telephone (in working order), a vending machine (stocked with food and drink) and a change machine (with change in it). Toilets should be nearby, and chairs should be comfortable and furniture attractive. Steps should be taken, as far as possible, to avoid using fixtures and fittings that could be used as weapons in an aggressive encounter. In ward areas, facilities may also be lacking because there are no arrangements for patients to help themselves to beverages, etc. Always having to ask staff for permission to make a drink causes immense frustration, especially if the request is denied or one is made to wait. Careful thought needs to be given to the likely effects of denying such basic freedoms. Staff are sometimes complacent about the impact on the patient of 'the rules', 'the ward routine' and the structure of the day in general. For those of us who can leave such constraints behind at the end of the shift, it is easy to forget the patient's perspective.

Another untoward environmental effect occurs where the general fabric and condition of a care setting is poor. This may engender a feeling that *people* are not cared for either, and patients may be more likely to damage property in such surroundings. Broken furniture should be repaired or replaced promptly, and the building should be kept in good order. A clean, well-kept surrounding invites favourable impressions. It has been our experience that staff who have been working in run-down conditions eventually tend not to notice the environment and accept it as it is. Continued working under such conditions may result in staff accepting generally low standards of nursing care, which, in more conducive surroundings, would be viewed as less than professional. We have also seen a state of hopelessness develop when staff attempts to alter the environment have been met by resistance because of inadequate funds and lack of management support.

There are a number of ways in which the environment can continue its assault on the senses. Noise can easily intrude, but, when little can be done to lessen the source, people can sometimes be distracted from the noise. Waiting rooms can be improved by the provision of reading material (regularly updated) and interesting objects, such as plants, pictures or an aquarium. Play areas where children can be seen should be provided. Television and video can also help to relieve the boredom of a long wait (Gillespie and Orton, 1985). Information about the hospital or clinic, including a 'who's who' of the staff and an outline of their work, might help to create a welcoming atmosphere and reduce anxiety, but some care must be taken with the tenor of the communications in case they are taken to be an affirmation of staff control. Bold notices, particularly those that appear to restrict activity, i.e. the 'Do Not' type, may be seen as provocative. In environments where smoking is banned, there is a case for saying that an area where smoking is permitted should be identified. A final sensory trigger to mention is that of odours, which, it has been argued, can be very distressing (Weitz, 1979). Staff sometimes become accustomed to the smells in their work environment, so they do not appreciate how unpleasant it may be for others, whereas for patients they may spark off a range of upsetting thoughts.

Leaving aside the obvious physical elements in an environment, it is sometimes the feelings evoked by the very idea of being in a hospital that can lead eventually to an individual's behaving aggressively. Patients often feel very vulnerable when first admitted to hospital. Reception areas, in particular, may be the scene of aggression. Overstressed staff may seem unsympathetic or brusque, or aggressive behaviour may arise because there is a lack of privacy afforded when discussing personal information; insensitive handling at this time can elicit an overreaction. It may also be prudent to consider the nature of nursing interactions. Although any nurse–patient interaction can result in aggression, it may be more likely during interactions that involve giving unwelcome information, carrying out painful procedures, the use of unfamiliar and 'frightening' machines or instruments, restricting another's liberty or deprivations of some sort (for instance, getting someone up when they would rather stay in bed). The recipe for safety in such situations may be very simple: by letting the patient know in good time of procedures to come staff can help him or her to understand what is happening and why, thus avoiding misinterpretation of nursing actions.

We end this chapter with a reminder that it is sometimes difficult to find any explanation for a hostile reaction. This may be because such reactions are often the result of an accumulation of minor irritations (socio-environmental influences) coming together in an individual already vulnerable due to illness and/or anxiety. Of course, nurses cannot be expected to guarantee stress-free environments for their patients. The nature of illness and the often unpleasant procedures nurses have to perform are likely to increase patients' fears and encourage aggression. However, we can strive to maintain an environment which is therapeutic, and we can alleviate the danger to ourselves and our charges by improving our awareness of the various influences that can contribute to aggression.

Further Reading

In the first two articles below the authors provide graphic accounts of how the combination of staff behaviour and the routines of hospital life interfere with appreciating the needs of patients.

Ford A (1990) Patients are worms. *Nursing Times*, **86** (15): 59.
Morrison A (1990) In a minute . . . *Nursing Times*, **86** (28): 41.
Morgan M (1986) Hospitals and patients. In Patrick D I and Scambler G (eds), *Sociology as Applied to Medicine*, chapter 6. Eastbourne: Baillière Tindall. (Looks at how staff attitudes and different care practices can influence staff–patient relationships.)

4
Factors Predisposing to Aggression

Key Points

- For some people, aggressive behaviour has previously been exhibited, and this could indicate a greater likelihood of its repetition.

- Staff must be informed when a patient is known to be aggressive.

- Consideration of factors both inside and outside the individual may help staff to take steps to avoid the problems of aggression.

- The nurse–patient relationship produces knowledge of the patient as a person and should be fostered as soon as the patient comes under care.

Causes of aggression may appear to originate from within the person as well as from outside. This means that an incident can occur without warning or any obvious reason, and this may be difficult to prepare for. For some people, reacting aggressively is a frequent occurrence, so it could be said to be reasonable to take past aggression as an important predictor that this behaviour will recur (Tupin, 1975). These people may use aggression for several reasons: it may be a form of manipulation they use to achieve some goal; it may be a habitual response to frustration, the person lacking other strategies for coping when faced with adversity; or it may simply be the person's regular mode of communication in the absence of more acceptable communication skills. Such behaviour can be seen as part of such a person's personality, and it is imperative that all staff are made aware of those who have been known to be aggressive. Student nurses on a new placement, in particular, should be given consideration, and when they are initially made aware of the situation, their requirements for support can be identified and explored. They should be given the opportunity to observe more experienced staff interacting with these patients, thereby increasing the students' confidence and skill for future interactions (Farrell, 1989). Learning on the job is vital if junior staff are to develop effective skills and attitudes.

However, there can be dangers in thinking about individuals in general terms, such as 'aggressive', as labels tend to cover up the other factors (both positive and negative) that make up a person. Once applied, labels become sticky and are difficult to shake off (Rosenhan, 1973; Sugden, 1985). When a nurse supposes that someone might be aggressive, he or she may unwittingly behave in a way (perhaps simply an unfriendly way) that provokes the very aggression that the nurse is seeking to avoid. It is often the new and inexperienced members of the team who are more vulnerable in these circumstances.

Try this exercise.

ACTIVITY 4

Write down examples from your own experience of causes of aggression that seem to have originated from within the individual.

Now see the discussion below.

Discussion
Firstly, it should not be assumed that aggression is more likely in someone who is mentally disordered. It is possible that those without any form of mental disorder account for the majority of incidents in all health care settings. This suggests the importance of 'everyday' factors in explaining why aggression has occurred, and these are discussed first here.

A number of factors predisposing an individual to behave aggressively stem simply from stress. Most people will react to illness itself with a stress reaction, the outward signs of which can be extremely varied, but suffice it to say that anyone might behave 'out of character' as a result of illness. Stress may make some people less tolerant, and it may interfere with judgement or perception, which can increase the risk of aggressive behaviour. Frequently, the stress of illness is heightened by fear. It should be noted that patients may have a wide range of fears. Volicer and Bohannon (1974) devised a scale to measure sources of in-patient stress. Among the most stressful experiences mentioned by patients were: the possibility of loss of function of the senses; admission for life-threatening illness; the possibility of loss of an organ; anticipation of bad experiences with medication; the possibility of disfigurement, an anticipated future loss of income; inadequate explanation of treatment; and the unconcerned attitude of staff. The least we should understand from these findings is that professionals do not always make the correct assumptions about what concerns the patient, which is desirable if steps are to be taken to create a therapeutic milieu.

There may also be even more deep-rooted reasons for aggression. It has been suggested that some patients feel they have been unjustly afflicted by their illness. They see themselves as a 'good person' and fail to understand the reasons for their condition. A range of emotions may be experienced, including depression, fear and anger (which may range from annoyance to bitter rebellion (Travelbee, 1976)). People may also be aggressive when they feel guilty about another person's injury. The parent of a child who has been injured because he or she has been poorly supervised while playing, for example, may react aggressively towards staff.

It was noted above that the presence of mental disorder in an individual should not be taken to mean that aggressive behaviour is any more likely, but it makes sense to exercise some caution in such a case, especially where the patient is not known to the staff. Aggression *may* occur in any form of mental illness. Paranoid illness, for example, could produce someone who firmly believes others are plotting to harm him or her, with the results that the patient reacts violently in 'self-defence'.

Many physical illnesses may themselves contribute to aggressiveness and, equally, should elicit a therapeutic management approach. Pain, diabetic reactions, cerebrovascular accidents and drug reactions may all predispose to aggressive behaviour, and, to complicate matters further, patients may present with a combination of factors that can mask the real reason for their aggression: 'The drunken, abusive patient's aggression may have little to do with his intake of alcohol; his fractured skull and raised intracranial pressure may also explain his behaviour' (Wright, 1989). Alcohol is certainly involved in many cases of aggression, especially those seen in the Accident and Emergency Department. This may sometimes be due largely to alcohol's so-called disinhibiting effects, but, subsequent to admission, alcohol may have other influences. Being in hospital often necessitates patients 'giving up' alcohol (or indeed smoking), which can result in withdrawal symptoms, of which increased irritability may be one. Feldman et al (1987) found, among a sample of 453 medical in-patients, that 18% of the men and 4% of the women admitted to having a drink problem, so this area should, perhaps, be explored if necessary.

Age can also be an important factor in episodes of aggression. Sometimes, young people have not developed sufficient control over their behaviour to cope with a difficult situation without using aggression. The elderly person may become disinhibited as a result of confusion. Feldman et al (1987) also found that 31% of medical in-patients over 70 years of age suffered from some kind of organic psychiatric disorder, possibly suggesting that at least the potential for aggression was high in the elderly.

There are certainly other internal factors giving rise to aggression, but it has not been an aim of this section to present a definitive list. Instead, it is intended that readers will be alerted to the possibility that such factors exist. Furthermore, where they do exist, they often operate in the background and may even be denied by the patient (Nichols, 1984). It is also intended that the discussion above will begin to help readers to get in touch with the emotions engendered in them by aggression caused in these ways. It is ironic that popular patients are identified as cheerful, quiet and undemanding (Stockwell, 1972), a tall order, perhaps, when one is ill!

INTERDEPENDENCY OF PRECIPITATING AND PREDISPOSING FACTORS

A distinction between internal and external causes of aggression has been drawn largely to highlight the existence of each. In any aggressive situation, however, it may be preferable to regard causation as the result of an interplay between the two. This chapter concludes by describing some of the ways in which they interrelate.

An important contribution to our understanding of aggressive responses comes from 'analysing', as far as possible, a patient's internal experiences and mental reactions to external events. The idea here is that it is not outside events *per se* but rather the patient's expectations and interpretations of events that are responsible for producing angry feelings (as well as anxiety, depression and other emotional states). It is often said that each individual is unique, and this helps to explain why people differ in their reactions to the same event. Take, for example, the reactions of non-smokers towards smokers. Some non-smokers are tolerant, while others are hostile. The self-talk of the tolerant might sound something like this: 'It's up to him what he does.

Who am I to say what's acceptable behaviour? Anyway he'll be gone soon'. The self-talk of the intolerant person may be: 'Why should I have to suffer his nasty habit? Who does he think he is polluting my air? He needs to be taught a lesson'. Of course, for most of us, there will be mitigating factors that help to control overreaction; for example, one might be very fond of the smoker even though his smoking is unpleasant. Sometimes we are unaware of our self-talk, and we interpret our angry feelings as being caused by the external event – 'Smoking in public makes me angry' – without acknowledging our own involvement, via anger-inducing self-talk, in the production of our anger. Establishing the nature of one's self-talk when angry should, therefore, form an important part of anger control training programmes, which are discussed on pages 74–5.

The interdependency of precipitating and predisposing factors in aggression in a health care context could be illustrated in the following example:

> A man who is under the influence of alcohol is admitted to hospital. He is kept waiting for some time, with no explanation, before being seen by a nurse. He demands to be seen. A nurse at the end of a long day responds with, 'Can't you see we're busy? You'll just have to wait your turn like everyone else'. The man feels slighted and responds with insults and gesticulations. The nurse becomes frightened and calls for help to control him.

Important factors here are: fear of the unknown effects of illness; the potential disruption that illness may cause to the man's daily routine; the disinhibiting effects of alcohol; having to wait without reason; the nurse's demeanour and response; the nurse's attitudes to people who are ill or injured following 'carelessness'; and the nurse's previous experience of patients affected by alcohol. Overwork, tiredness and feeling easily annoyed should be seen as signals to oneself to take action to lessen the likelihood of overreacting to the everyday demands of the job.

The interaction between the roles of the self, the other person and the environment in bringing about aggression is illustrated in this example and summarised in Figure 4.1. These three elements form the foundations on which *proactive* interventions can be built. Where staff are more aware of the roles of each element, they will be able to take steps to reduce the likelihood of aggression. Proactive responses should start even before patients come under the nurse's care. Each setting will have different requirements, and these must be ascertained and discussed at unit level.

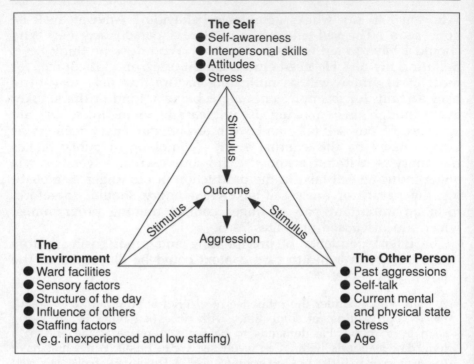

Fig 4.1   Factors influencing aggression: the health care context

Nurses in the Accident and Emergency Department, for example, may decide that more could be done to meet the needs of people waiting to be seen – needs for information about waiting times, perhaps. Ward staff might consider ways to improve the admitting nurse's knowledge of a new patient before his or her arrival. For in-patients, fostering open communication between staff and patients may enable staff to identify those people with aggression simmering beneath the surface.

Communication skills almost always prove to be the key to therapeutic management in aggression, and this is emphasised here. All nurse–patient interactions should be seen as opportunities for communication. However, patients are unlikely to say very much in interactions that are short, lack privacy or have the completion of a task as their main focus. Also, if nurses are perceived to be very busy, patients will be reluctant to 'disturb' them. To encourage patient communication, we must show that we are available and willing to talk. Communicating our availability requires a verbal indication – 'Is there anything else I can help with?' – and, probably more importantly, actions that support the words, for example standing still instead of slowly withdrawing. Taking the time to chat to patients about everyday issues will also help. Although the pressures on nursing time make this difficult, regular contact such as this can enable a nurse to appreciate the patient as an individual and help guide interactions to pre-empt the triggers to aggression.

Good nurse–patient communication is important for another reason. Breakwell (1989) asserts:

> It is supremely ironic that most caring professions as a matter of course restrict the freedom and independence of the client . . . We are both agents of social control and facilitators of well-being.

In the nursing context, restriction of patient freedom can be seen in many situations: patients are confined to bed; access to information may be withheld; access to even basic amenities, for example, a bedpan may have to be requested; meal times are often fixed; visiting times may be restricted; and some patients may be in hospital against their will. Breakwell suggests that nurses have to negotiate a difficult path, which balances the profession's desire to respect the patient's wishes with the inherent restrictiveness of many aspects of nursing care. The patient has to balance the desire for expert care against the prospect of loss of personal control. Achieving the right balance is going to be more likely where there is an atmosphere that fosters two-way communication, so that nurses have a chance of eliciting factors that may bring about aggression. Awareness of the interdependency of precipitating and predisposing factors forms the basis for demonstrating proactive intervention.

Further Reading

Beck A T (1976) *Cognitive Therapy and the Emotional Disorders*. New York: International Universities Press. (A very readable account of the relationship between thoughts and emotions.)

French P (1983) *Social Skills for Nursing Practice*. London: Croom Helm. (Chapter 4 provides a useful introduction to interview skills in the nursing context.)

Ley P (1988) *Communicating with Patients: Improving Communication, Satisfaction and Compliance*. London: Croom Helm. (Offers suggestions for improving nurse–patient communication and is one of the few books that reviews non-compliance among health care professionals as well as among patients.)

Part II

RELATE

It is assumed that where staff are more aware of the possible causes of aggression, its incidence may be reduced because preventive measures are possible. Part II considers the staff responses necessary where prevention has not been possible or effective and aggression is a reality. Because of the prolonged time which nurses spend in contact with patients, they have the highest risk of any of the disciplines of encountering aggression, and few nursing contexts escape the chances of aggression completely. The keyword in Part II is RELATE, referring to the need to relate therapeutically to people displaying aggressive behaviour. For this to be possible, the nurse must have high-level interpersonal skills and, for those occasions when physical intervention is required, expert techniques in physical control. It is sometimes thought that the use of physical control denotes failure or even a total lack of interpersonal skills, but it is argued that the two types of skill should be seen as complementary.

5
Recognising Verbal and Non-verbal Signs of Aggression

Key Points

- People vary in the way in which they express aggression.

- Knowing the patient well enables the nurse to notice the changes that signal aggression for a particular patient.

- The likelihood of aggression may be increased during the early development of a close relationship.

- If nurses are to resist stress, they need to develop characteristics that enable them to be effective practitioners.

It is our experience that patient aggression rarely occurs without warning signs of some kind. Nurses need to develop high-level skills of observation and recognition of impending aggression. In practice, the experience of nursing aggressive patients enables many nurses to become acutely sensitive to the indicators, especially if there is 'in-service' training in support. In units where aggression rarely occurs, staff do not get this experience, and their preparation for aggression needs to be approached differently. However, all nurses should heed the 'feeling' that a patient is growing aggressive, as a situation can get out of hand if intuitive 'warning signs' are ignored. Gorski and Miller (1981) suggest:

> always listen to your stomach: a strange feeling in the pit of your stomach is a sign that you should begin looking to the patient to see if there are some cues or messages that may be indicating the potential for aggression.

Check your senses, even the olfactory one, as there is some evidence to suggest that there is such a thing as 'a smell of anger' (Wiener, 1979). REMEMBER, *if you feel frightened report it*.

Try this exercise.

ACTIVITY 5

Think about the last time you encountered aggressive behaviour in an individual. Did you notice any changes in his or her behaviour before the incident? Try to remember if there were any changes in *your* verbal and non-verbal behaviour in response to your feelings.

Now see the discussion below.

Discussion

Listed below are the responses given by a group of student nurses when asked: 'What do you do when you get angry?':

Swear	Go red in the face
Shout	Complain to someone else
Throw things	Kick the dog
Sulk	Tap my fingers
Cry	Become sarcastic
Smash things up	Violent exercises
Go to bed	Glare
Go for a walk	Stammer
Run out and slam the door	Go silent
Argue	

The above list begins to indicate the variety of behaviours that may forewarn of aggression. It neatly highlights verbal and non-verbal, inwardly-directed and outwardly-directed, acceptable and unacceptable behaviours. Some of these would be obvious, others less so. Sometimes 'everyday' communications become signals of aggression when they are accompanied by changes in voice pitch and tone, when the speed of the utterance is unusual or when they are supported by particular facial expressions. These signs may pass rapidly in practice and, unfortunately, there is often little time to reflect on their significance, yet they can reveal important clues to future behaviours. Recognition of anger in a patient indicates the need for the nurse to proceed with caution in the interaction. It is also useful to acknowledge one's own responses when faced with aggressive behaviour, as these provide cues. Sometimes one's own autonomic changes, palpitations for example, are the first sign of impending aggression. It is important to be aware of these phenomena because it seems it may be best that some patients do not realise that staff can be afraid; looking composed and confident conveys an idea that the nurse remains a steadying influence for someone who is out of control. One's own outward appearance when faced with aggression certainly needs to be thought about and may need to be 'improved'.

Many people adopt a particular behaviour when angry, as the student nurses' responses above seem to show. This knowledge may help to heighten one's awareness of the potential for aggression in an encounter, but it would be a mistake to think that people have a set way of behaving in all situations. Our everyday observations tell us that the way we express our anger at home may be quite different from the way we feel we can do so at work. However, the experienced nurse does not leave all to chance. Often the clue to impending aggression is not so much in the type of behaviour seen but rather in the fact that the person's current behaviour changes, so that a calm person become agitated, a noisy person becomes quiet and a quiet person becomes loud, or perhaps even more quiet! It is, therefore, important that nurses get to know their patients as individuals whenever possible. The trust and understanding on which the nurse–patient relationship is built enables the patient to voice his or her fears and anxieties.

In units where there is a rapid turnover of patients, as in Accident and Emergency Departments, nurses will rarely have the time to get to know their patients well. In these circumstances, one needs even greater sensitivity to the early indicators of potential aggression. Furthermore, nurses in these settings often need to decide *quickly* whether or not a patient is angry. Needless to say, we suggest erring on the side of caution. In momentarily mistaking the patient's screwed up face as an expression of anger instead of pain, it is unlikely that any harm will be done. A friendly enquiry at a safe distance will not go amiss when this happens. In situations where there is greater opportunity to spend time with patients, primary nursing offers nurses the opportunity to give high-quality care based on a knowledge of the patient's individual needs and difficulties. Whenever possible, the primary nurse personally administers the care, thereby increasing his or her knowledge of the patient as a person. This is in contrast to traditional, task-orientated care in which relationships, and thus knowledge of the patient, are probably more superficial.

However, the formation of a close relationship may, in the early stages, increase the likelihood of patient aggression. The nurse may be seen as an authority figure or the patient may test the strength of the nurse's concern for him or her by trying to provoke an aggressive response in the nurse. Lyttle (1986) reminds us that:

the therapeutic nurse–patient relationship does not suppress or censor expressions of aggression; it accepts them, explores them, tries to heighten the patient's awareness of the reasons for them and provides constructive channels for them, for example, assisting the patient to express anger verbally rather than through physical assault.

Responding to distressed and aggressive patients can put heavy demands on the nurse, and some resilience is necessary if he or she is not to succumb to these pressures. To continue to be an effective practitioner in the face of aggression, the nurse should attempt to cultivate certain characteristics. Brammer (1979) suggests that the presence of the following six characteristics are important for helping another person.

1. *An awareness of self and values.* The suggestion here is that we need to be self-aware of a wide range of issues so that we can answer such questions as 'Who am I?' and 'What is important to me?' Many of our interactions with patients will test and challenge our own views and values, so it is important that we are fairly clear in our own minds what we believe is important, while at the same time accepting other people's views.
2. *The ability to analyse one's own feelings.* This is a necessary attribute if we are to avoid 'countertransference effects', i.e. the unconscious transfer of feelings one has towards people in the past onto the patient. Such transfer of feelings may include rejection, indulgence, overprotection, domination and love.
3. *The ability to serve as a model and influencer.* We cannot avoid being seen as influencers of and models for our patients. For some nurses, being a role model means being 'yourself' with patients at all times, i.e. behaving towards patients as one would with a friend. However, our view is that for most of us, being 'yourself' in the face of aggression is far from satisfactory. We believe that if nurses are to relate therapeutically to aggressive clients, the skills required have first to be learned in order to *become* 'natural' responses.
4. *Altruism, or a strong commitment to the other that transcends concerns for material rewards.* In the nursing context, altruistic behaviour can be seen in small acts such as allowing the elderly patient that little bit of extra time to move in bed, anticipating the patient's need for a cool drink, staying close to a distressed patient and allowing an angry patient time to vent his or her views. However, it is worth considering that our wish to help another is also fulfilling needs for ourselves, for example of self-esteem, social acceptance and feeling

wanted. Careful consideration of our motives is essential in this area if we are to avoid acting blindly, and possibly destructively, in our relationships with our patients.

5. *A strong sense of ethics.*   We should be committed to upholding standards of patient care that are in keeping with our own views and those of the profession and society.
6. *Responsibility.*   This relates to an awareness of how much we, as helpers, have responsibility for another person. Do we, for example, know our own limitations? Are we clear where our responsibilities lie in relation to the help we offer to patients?

There are numerous ways in which the characteristics outlined above can be developed, as the following examples suggest. Firstly, take time to reflect on your beliefs and past behaviour; this may be carried out alone or with a trusted friend. Secondly, form an ongoing quality circle group where patient care issues are discussed and evaluated. Thirdly, ask for supervisory sessions. In an ideal situation one should discuss one's practice with a mentor who has experience in supervision. Fourthly, request feedback from colleagues and maybe even patients; this could be centred on such issues as your performance in certain situations or patient satisfaction. Fifthly, attend study days and workshops. These have two important uses: they allow participants to reassess their views and skills and acquire some new ones; and they afford a break from the demands of the job – getting away from the work situation to meet colleagues and share experiences can be just as important in re-energising oneself as can the acquisition of new skills.

The integrity of the effective helper (nurse) is vital if therapeutic management of aggression is valued. Increasing self-awareness helps to improve skills, enables skill deficits to be identified and gives one the ability to ask for help when necessary. If personal knowledge of the patient is added to the equation, we will have done everything possible to reduce the likelihood and minimise the effects of aggression.

Further Reading

Manthey M (1980) *The Practice of Primary Nursing.* Boston: Blackwell Scientific Publications. (A standard text, but orientated towards general hospital nursing.)

Morris D (1977) *Manwatching: A Field Guide to Human Behaviour.* London: Jonathan Cape. (A very accessible and popularised insight into the role of gesture and other non-verbal behaviours in communication.)

6
Making Therapeutic Responses to Aggression

Key Points

- Manner and outward appearance play a major role in the management of aggression.

- A nurse's underlying emotional state may leak out.

- 'Talking over' is an alternative to meeting force with force.

- People who use aggression frequently in everyday relationships may benefit from specific long-term help.

- Limit setting can be used when other interventions have failed.

- A united, consistent staff approach is essential.

- Nurses should consider their own personal safety if aggression seems likely.

- All staff should know how to summon help.

- Restraint should only be used if other measures are inappropriate, and should not be carried out alone.

- Do not forget bystanders: they may be frightened or want to help out.

- Inappropriate use of mechanical restraint and sedative drugs may amount to a form of patient abuse.

- Seclusion must be used appropriately.

In managing aggression remember to attend to
Self-presentation
otherwise
Self-preservation
may become your priority.

SELF-PRESENTATION

What you say and what you do are important in determining the outcome of any interaction involving aggression. For example, looking tough and answering back can escalate the encounter. Your own non-verbal communication may be a very important instrument in dealing with aggression. The following approaches to engagement should be considered:

- Appear confident and concerned.
- Don't overreact.
- Avoid getting into arguments.
- Don't take abuse personally.
- Be consistent in your approach.
- Monitor your performance – ask yourself, 'How am I doing? Am I making matters worse?' Think about how you might be coming across to the other person. For example, is your tone of voice soft and reassuring? Are you standing at the right distance? Between 9 ft and 12 ft is felt to be an appropriate distance for professionals to interact with clients (Hall, 1959, in Hargie et al, 1987). Are you looking at the other when spoken to? Are your hands visible? Is your posture generally open and relaxed? As Abercrombie (1968) says, 'We speak with our vocal organs, but we converse with our whole body'.

Try this exercise.

ACTIVITY 6

It is often difficult in aggressive encounters to remain completely calm and composed. As a consequence, your underlying emotional state may 'leak out', for example by you clenching your fists. What leaks have you noticed in others or in yourself?
  Now see the discussion below.

Discussion
The expression of aggression is often the result of conflict between, on the one hand, the basic physiological and emotional need to express aggression and, on the other hand, our conscious attempts to conceal it. We are continually faced with situations in which we get angry or annoyed but are reluctant to say how we feel for fear of the consequences. For example, your boss may irritate you, but telling him or her so may lead to you losing your job. But what happens to anger that is controlled or damped down? Does it just fade away? Experience tells us that this

sometimes happens. What was irritating the night before may appear insignificant the next day. However, in contrast, anger may sometimes be kept 'on hold', to be released at a later time, as any domestic cat can testify! Experience also suggests that it is not always easy to put anger on hold without some part of it showing through. These 'leaks' can occur during the anger-provoking incident and/or at some time later. Furthermore, for some of us the 'leaks' may endure for a long time – for weeks or even years after the event.

Evidence of underlying anger may appear as:

- slips of the tongue;
- rapid speech;
- altered tone of voice;
- interruptions;
- put downs, e.g. 'God knows, John tries, don't you dear.' Or 'Janet, dear, perhaps you could ask Margaret how she manages to make such beautiful coffee'. Or 'You know, Alan is so good around the house I sometimes wonder if he's in the wrong job';
- disagreements, e.g. 'I hear what you say, but with the greatest respect, Mr Smith . . .';
- self-deprecations;
- pulling rank;
- nail biting;
- handling patients roughly;
- ignoring patients' needs;
- being unduly prejudiced;
- complaining;
- scapegoating;
- accident proneness;
- driving too fast;
- posture shifts, e.g. arms folded, head back;
- indigestion, red face, skin disorders and a range of other physical manifestations, which may be indicative of an underlying aggressive and anxious state (Salkovskis, 1989).

SELF-PRESERVATION

In aggressive encounters, most people fear for their personal safety, yet lack of forethought can provoke the very hostility one wants to avoid. Consider the situation where a patient is refused access to the kitchen, 'until it is time for tea'. The patient then ignores the nurse and proceeds to enter the kitchen. The nurse rebukes the patient. The patient hits out at the nurse. Attempts to dissuade the patient by physical intervention only increase his resolve to make his cup of tea. Remember, it is seldom wise to try to restrain someone single-handedly, particularly in situations where there is only minor 'offence'. In this scenario, the nurse may see her refusal of the patient's request as causing only minor inconvenience. To a patient, whose life revolves around certain routines, such refusal may be viewed as the final straw in an environment filled with oppression.

There are ways of coping with aggression that minimise the threat to self through verbal means while avoiding overreaction; this is what would be necessary in the above example. Such verbal means are, in this text, termed 'talking over', one aim of which is that it should encourage us to think about the other person's perspective before making a response. Essentially, talking over involves calming aggressive behaviour by use of verbal responses. It is intended as an alternative to meeting force with force. Where talking over is accompanied by an attempt to understand the patient's needs, the nurse fosters conciliation. The underlying rationale for talking over is that talking helps – *Better to talk it out than fight it out*.

These points are illustrated in the examples that follow. Make your own response before looking at the possible responses on pages 59–66.

1. A woman you spoke to about her problems now states angrily, 'It's your fault I'm upset. Go away. You don't know how to help me. I hate you'.
2. A man who has been kept waiting for his tablets shouts, 'Hurry up, will you? I want my tablets **now**'.
3. A man who has been drinking arrives on the unit late at night and states, 'I'm staying until I've seen a doctor'. (He refuses to say why he wants a doctor.)
4. A woman who believes people are plotting against her says sharply, 'You are talking about me. I know you want to kill me'.
5. A young man, when asked how he is by a student nurse who is new to the ward, replies, 'Fuck off. Leave me alone'.
6. A man who has been in hospital for several years paces the floor while shouting and gesticulating at passers by.
7. Two loud and drunk youths arrive in Accident and Emergency late at night. One of the youths is bleeding from a cut hand, the other demands help for his 'injured mate'. When you arrive to investigate, they offer you a can of beer, saying,

'Have a drink with us girl, you look as if you could do with a couple of nice blokes like us'.

8. On a home visit, a patient accuses you of interfering. When you attempt to leave, he threatens to hit you unless you stay and 'hear him out'. You are aware that this patient has assaulted nurses and others in the past.

9. A patient's daughter continuously asserts that her father's care is inadequate, despite reassurance to the contrary (no evidence has ever arisen to suggest ill treatment). She is very critical of all aspects of care. For example, she regularly accuses the staff of losing her father's clothes and neglecting his personal hygiene. She is a tall, well-built lady and adopts a very intimidating posture – she stands with her hands on her hips and points with her finger. When irate, she stands very close and pokes the nurse on the chest. Her father is admitted for respite care on a regular basis. He suffers from aphasia and has a hemiplegia of several years' standing. She comes into the ward office and angrily states, 'What have you done with Dad's new set of dentures? And his hair is not combed; he's got dirty fingers, wet shoes and a runny nose.'

Possible Responses

1. *A woman you spoke to about her problems now states angrily, 'It's your fault I'm upset. Go away. You don't know how to help me. I hate you'.*

Such remarks can be hurtful, leading to an almost instant reaction of resentment with a desire to save face. But reflect on the situation for a moment. Use a response that might help you understand why the woman is reacting in this way. Is it really that she hates you or is it that she is upset and embarrassed after telling you about her problems? Be ready to try to understand the situation that is facing you. A response that focuses attention on to the woman might be appropriate here. For example, you might say, 'You sound very upset with me'. Pause and wait for her response. Simply reflecting back what she seems to be feeling may help her to locate more clearly the source of her discomfort or hostility and facilitate discussion. See Chapter 3 in Nelson-Jones (1983) for more information on the use of reflection in counselling.

2. *A man who has been kept waiting for his tablets shouts, 'Hurry up, will you? I want my tablets now'.*

The response here is to accept that the man has a reason to be upset. An apology might be in order here: 'I'm sorry that you have been kept waiting. I expect you thought we'd forgotten you.

I'll get your tablets now'. Often, it is important not just to apologise but to acknowledge what the person might be thinking and/or feeling. In this case, the man might have felt ignored. Ohbuchi et al (1989) found that when an apology was given to undergraduate students who had previously been given unwarranted negative evaluations, they were less likely to respond with aggression when compared to students who had not received an apology.

3.   *A man who has been drinking arrives on the unit late at night and states, 'I'm staying until I've seen a doctor'. (He refuses to say why he wants a doctor.)*

Although it would be unwise to confront him with the unreasonable nature of his behaviour, it is important to accept that he is concerned about something. The verbal response might be, 'Come and have a cup of tea and I'll see if a doctor is available'. This will, at least, give you a 'breathing space' to decide on your next move: you might want to get non-medical help or you may decide that it is appropriate to get the doctor.

4.   *A woman who believes people are plotting against her says sharply, 'You are talking about me. I know you want to kill me'.*

First consider what this woman may be feeling and thinking. Ask yourself, 'What can I say that is likely to reassure her that I am not out to harm her and to help her to talk further about her fears?' The person with paranoid thinking often feels insecure and lacks self-esteem, and the more threatened the person feels, the greater the feelings of personal insecurity. Such feelings are too painful for the person to acknowledge consciously, and instead the defence mechanism of projection is used. Blaming and accusing others serves to protect the person from acknowledging the reality of his or her circumstances.

This is a tricky situation to respond to. To insist that you are not out to harm her may serve only to convince her that, in fact, you are. Further, to tell someone you will do no harm may sow a seed of doubt in the person's mind that you *could* if you wanted to. A response here might be to say, 'I wish you well [woman's name]. It must be very worrying for you believing this.' Pause, wait for a response. Allow the lady to set her own pace. Give her the right to complain. Listen calmly and respectfully. It might be appropriate to follow up this lady's response with, 'What is it that causes you to believe this?', or 'Is there anything I can do to show you that you are safe with us?' This will pave the way for further discussion. The goal is to help this lady to feel accepted and as secure as possible. Do not try to convince her through logical reasoning of her mistaken belief. A suspicious person will cling even more tenaciously to a belief if feeling threatened by appeals to reason. Avoid reinforcing any delusional verbalisations; talk about the rational aspects of the conversation. If the patient continues to misinterpret the reality of the situation, you should tactfully discontinue the interaction by making it clear you are not rejecting her but rather the delusional verbalisation (Lyttle 1986). You might say, 'It's difficult for me to understand you at this moment. Maybe we could talk again later?' Whenever the patient does converse rationally, reinforce her, saying, 'I like it when we can talk like this'. A consistent, non-defensive response is required, together with a willingness to look behind the patient's words – feeling so important that others might want to kill her may be hiding feelings of insignificance, although, of course, it would be unwise to suggest this to the patient. Stripping away such defences is likely to increase the person's anxiety even further. It is better to help the person feel safe, as it is only when she feels secure that she can begin to think about alternative ways of relating to you.

5.   *A young man, when asked how he is by a student nurse who is new to the ward replies, 'Fuck off. Leave me alone'.*

A response here might be, 'You want to be left alone now. I'll come back later'. With this response, the man's wish to be left alone is acted upon but an opening is left for a later meeting. Note the cue that things are not all right. Observe unobtrusively, and forewarn colleagues.

6.   *A man who has been in hospital for several years paces the floor while shouting and gesticulating at passers by.*

Ask yourself, 'How well do I know this man. How will he react to me?' If you are not very familiar with the patient, enlist the help of another who knows the man well, as this will help to predict the likely outcome of particular interventions. In this situation, the man may be willing to talk about his favourite topic to someone he knows well.

7.   *Two loud and drunk youths arrive in Accident and Emergency late at night. One of the youths is bleeding from a cut hand, the other demands help for his 'injured mate'. When you arrive to investigate, they offer you a can of beer, saying, 'Have a drink with us girl, you look as if you could do with a couple of nice blokes like us'.*

To begin with, consider how these youths might be feeling. There may well be fear and anxiety beneath the numbed exterior created by the alcohol, and these feelings may need to be acknowledged. Furthermore, try to decide what kind of roles are being adopted; one at least sounds rather 'macho'. In situations like this, with sexual overtones, where there is a drunken male striving for dominance, it might be as well to treat the remarks as representing a friendly gesture from one who has limited social skills. A smile, taking care not to condone any of the sexual intent in the youths' message, and a reply such as, 'The important thing right now is for you to help me see what's wrong with that hand' may help to distract attention away from you. With some drunks, the most effective ploy may be to humour them, although one must be clear of the dividing line between that and something like sarcasm which may seem provocative.

Next you should take the initiative. Say how you would like to go about your assessment of the injury, and if possible enlist the help of the uninjured man; perhaps he could assist by removing his friend's coat. Explain the likely procedure to come and if you need to take the patient away for treatment, keep the other person informed of what is happening. At this stage, remember once more the likely feelings of the injured party as he is being treated. Talk to him. Explain in simple language what you are about to do. If the treatment is going to hurt, inform the patient of this and suggest things he can do to minimise the discomfort. Remember whether his friend was willing to be involved in a helping capacity; if he was uncooperative, it would be sensible to separate the two by simply asking the friend to leave.

Choosing a suitable strategy for responding to aggression in people who have been drinking is fraught with difficulty because many 'normal' interaction processes are disrupted by alcohol. An alternative approach where alcohol was not necessarily involved might have begun with a reply such as, 'No thanks. I'd like to get on with attending to your friend's hand'. Where the nurse feels sexually harassed, it is important that she sends a 'stop' message clearly early on in the interaction. Some responses that the nurse might make are: 'Please stop. I do not want you to hold me round the waist'; 'When you [describe the behaviour you want stopped], I feel uneasy and I want you to stop doing it'; 'Our working relationship is good, but I don't want any other sort of relationship with you'; 'When you [describe the person's behaviour], I get scared because I feel threatened'. In these encounters, it is particularly important that non-verbal behaviour echoes what is being said: there should be no discrepancy between what we say and how we say it. In other words, as Jesus of Nazareth said 2000 years ago, 'Let your eyes be a clear

"Yes", and your "No" no. Anything else spells trouble' (from *Matthew* 5:37 as cited in Bolton, 1986). Also, avoid the temptation of going overboard with your stop message as it may encourage an aggressive response in the receiver. Finally, resist the temptation to judge or make moralistic comments on the offending behaviour. It is best to confine descriptions to what the person does in terms of his or her behaviour. For example, drop the word 'pester' in the following response, 'When you pester me I . . .', in favour of 'When you continually ask me out I . . .'. In this way the person is left in no doubt about what behaviour you are referring to, and it is more difficult for the offender to sidestep the issue.

8.   *On a home visit, a patient accuses you of interfering. When you attempt to leave, he threatens to hit you unless you stay and 'hear him out'. You are aware that this person has assaulted nurses and others in the past.*

This is a potentially very dangerous situation and therefore requires you to remain composed while you reflect on how best to proceed. It is important that you stay calm, which essentially means controlling your anxiety. This can be achieved in several ways. Some people use self-statements, i.e. they silently say some word or phrase that helps them to relax, for instance 'This is going to be a difficult situation but I can handle it' or 'Let's take this one step at a time'. Control of muscle tension and breathing is another method of reducing anxiety. Gorski and Miller (1981) suggest that self-control can be achieved by paying attention to:

- *breathing* – breathe deeply, rhythmically and deliberately;
- *posture* – relax and evenly balance your weight for effective and rapid movement (see page 69);
- *thought patterns* – think realistically and optimistically about your situation, then divert your thoughts about yourself to the situation you are involved in;
- *emotional control* – accept as normal feelings of panic, anger and fear. Control these feelings by attention to breathing, posture and thought control;
- *behavioural control* – never be discouraged if you make a mistake in a crisis. No failure is final and no success is guaranteed. Be alert and do the best you know how.

Other possible reponses in this situation might be:

- Say you will stay but explain the need to phone your office to let them know where you are as you are expected back shortly (such calls to base may in fact be a coded message asking for help).

- Listen carefully to what the patient has to say while considering escape options should the situation be seen to be getting out of control.
- Use diversionary tactics. Talk about things that might be of particular interest to the man. Finney (1988) cites the case of a health visitor who, when confronted by the axe-wielding husband of a patient she went to visit, used diversionary tactics. The health visitor noticed voodoo artefacts in the room and began talking to the man about his voodoo practices. She was eventually allowed to leave.
- A combination of the above.

As far as possible try to normalise the situation. Consider sitting down, and invite the other person to do so too. You may even admit that you are scared and that you would find it easier to talk if you felt less threatened. This situation raises an important question: Why are you visiting this patient on your own in the first place, bearing in mind his violence to others in the past? Home visiting is made all the more risky when on your own. It may not always be practical to have two nurses visiting patients' homes, but in situations where patients have been aggressive in the past, there should be provision made so that employees are not placed in unnecessary danger. All community workers, whether alone or in pairs, should be aware of how help can be summoned in an emergency; this is followed up in Chapter 11.

9. *A patient's daughter continuously asserts that her father's care is inadequate, despite reassurance to the contrary (no evidence has ever arisen to suggest ill treatment). She is very critical of all aspects of care. For example, she regularly accuses the staff of losing her father's clothes and neglecting his personal hygiene. She is a tall, well-built lady and adopts a very intimidating posture – she stands with her hands on her hips and points with her finger. When irate, she stands very close and pokes the nurse on the chest. Her father is admitted for respite care on a regular basis. He suffers from aphasia and has a hemiplegia of several years' standing. She comes into the ward office and angrily states, 'What have you done with Dad's new set of dentures? And his hair is not combed; he's got dirty fingers, wet shoes and a runny nose.'*

Any suggestion of neglect is a sure way to hit a nurse's 'crumple button', and it is vital that you do not rise to the provocation. Firstly, invite this lady to sit down. Achieving this immediately removes her domineering stance. (You may have to sit first to encourage compliance.) Listen openly to the complaint and reassure her that you will investigate. Assuming that these current allegations are groundless, we suggest that you supportively confront this lady about her behaviour. The aim here is to seek an alternative avenue of communication in order to break the cycle of allegation–reassurance–allegation. There may be rational elements to her behaviour. For example, she may have very high standards, which are, in this case, too high for a hospital environment. She may also feel very guilty about leaving her father, and, perhaps, unconsciously displaces her concern onto you. She may also feel very vulnerable herself in the hospital context and lack the skills to control her anxiety.

Next, acknowledge that this lady is upset and that hospital is not like home. Leave other suspicions you might have concerning the underlying reasons for her behaviour until later. You have to bring her round, tactfully and gently, to exploring other issues below the surface. Timing here is crucial, and a premature comment will increase defensiveness.

Nurse Mrs Hatchett I can see that you are upset about your father. I'm, upset, too, when you believe we are not caring for him well. Of course, being in hospital is not the same as being in your own home. (*Pause, wait for the lady's response.*)

Note that in the above statement the nurse states that she, too, is upset, thus making it more difficult for Mrs Hatchett to complain about the nurse not being concerned. This will help to focus the issue on the difference between hospital and home, not on the difference between the nurse and the lady.

Mrs Hatchett This is my Dad we're talking about here. My Dad deserves the best.

Continue to acknowledge this lady's feelings. Remind her that you consider her father's hospital care to be very good. The idea here is that if you show clearly the impasse that has developed, she may be more willing to try an alternative avenue of relating to you.

Nurse Of course he does, and as we've already discussed, we feel that our present care is very good.

Mrs Hatchett Look at the state of him. Is that good care?

Nurse Yes, I know you feel upset, but we feel Harry's care is really very good.

Mrs Hatchett Well, you'll have to do better. My Dad deserves the best.

Nurse He does deserve the best. Harry's care is really very good. You know, Mrs Hatchett, I wonder if maybe there is something else we should be talking about to help resolve our differences.

Notice that the nurse does not discount Mrs Hatchett's views; she accepts that there is a difference of opinion. This is an important point. If you imply that you are right, you are, by implication, saying that she is wrong, and a power struggle develops. Notice also that the nurse 'acts like a politician' – she alters the basis of the argument – which shifts the focus away from the patient and onto Mrs Hatchett.

Mrs Hatchett   I don't know, you're the bloody nurse.

Nurse   Well, maybe it would help if we could have a chat about your father prior to his illness to help me understand a bit more how you feel.

Mrs Hatchett   Well, what do you want to know?

Now the nurse can begin to explore the reasons behind Mrs Hatchett's allegation and seek solutions through non-aggressive encounters.

Occasionally, nurses may be asked to fulfil 'impossible' requests, for example a patient may demand extra medication even though the doctor has refused any increase in the dosage. In such situations the 'two-step no' response may be appropriate. This assertion technique allows for refusal of the request while acknowledging the other's feelings and needs, thereby making it less likely that the other person will feel completely powerless in the situation. 'I think I can understand why you want more medication but the doctor is not going to prescribe it', would make the patient less likely to feel loss of dignity, feelings and power, and would pave the way for constructive discussion (Kaplan and Wheeler, 1983). In such situations, a flat 'no' can come across as aggressive, rejecting and uncaring.

Wondrak (1989) suggests that nurses need to develop a range of assertion techniques in response to patients' verbal abuse. He outlines five techniques based on the work of Smith (1975):

1. *Self disclosure*, for example admitting to the aggressor that you are afraid.
2. *Partial agreement.* Agreeing with part of the patient's criticism. Wondrak gives the following example. Person 1 – 'Just look at the way you dress'. Person 2 – 'Yes . . . you may be right there, the colours clash. I quite like the effect though'.
3. *Gentle confrontation.* Here the nurse supportively confronts the

other in an attempt to uncover the reason behind the abusive comments. For example, person 2 above could continue with, 'I'm not deliberately dressing to upset you. I can't help noticing that the way I dress seems to upset you'.

4. *Side stepping*, or agreeing fully with the other's criticism. Patient says, 'Fancy putting on a dressing like that'. Nurse says, 'Yes I agree, it is not a good job'.

5. *Being specific*, i.e. keeping what you have to say as specific as possible and avoiding unnecessary padding.

Assertiveness skills can help to diffuse an aggressive encounter or may, indeed, prevent such encounters ever arising. Kaplan and Wheeler (1983) suggest that passivity can invite aggression. The passive person is viewed as helpless and acceding to the threat. Many nurses feel it is uncaring to be assertive, believing that it is wrong to refuse requests or to communicate clearly and directly one's thoughts and feelings. At least two reasons may account for this view. Firstly, assertion is seen solely in terms of standing up for one's rights and the other crucial elements of assertion are ignored. Being assertive does not preclude the use of negotiating skills, which is an important consideration, particularly in the context of aggression. It is often very difficult to know when one's legitimate rights are, in fact, being usurped. Therefore, the nurse has to be prepared to offer a compromise so that the aggressor suffers minimal loss of face. Secondly, assertion is thought of as simply mastering a range of inter-personal techniques, and the intrapersonal dimension is ignored. Learning a range of assertion techniques is only half the requirement for *being* assertive. The other equally important ingredient is the development of an assertive attitude, which includes self-confidence based on a belief in one's own worth. It manifests itself in the ability to respect others' views without being deferential or feeling superior. The truly assertive person can express feelings of love, affection, admiration, approval and agreement, deal with criticism, confront others (supportively) and express feelings spontaneously (Gerry, 1989).

Finally, in an aggressive encounter, one can consider asking the person to leave and come back when he or she has 'cooled down'. This may be useful in situations where the nurse feels he or she can control the situation to a large extent, for example when dealing with children. The idea behind the 'time out' is that the person is given time for his or her arousal levels to subside, which may take up to 90 minutes (Kaplan and Wheeler, 1983). Provision of a 'neutral' environment, i.e. one that is not likely to foment anger, for the 'time out', will help in arousal reduction. The nurse may subject herself to a 'time out', too. For example, when a patient refuses a request, the nurse can offer to come back later, when he or she has had a chance to think about it. In this situation, 'time out' may offer a measure of face-saving on the part of the patient, who has the option to change his or her mind without coercion from the nurse.

Below are some points to bear in mind when 'talking over'.

- *Be supportive – avoid defensiveness.* Consider the feelings and thoughts of the aggressor. Accept that the other is angry and avoid retaliatory remarks. Ask questions that focus on the aggressor; for example, you might ask, 'How long have you been feeling like that?' rather than saying, 'I know just how you feel'. Be prepared to accept and even seek criticism. For example, you might ask the other person what it is about your behaviour that is annoying. Give him or her time and space to express thoughts and feelings and do not be in a hurry to resolve the encounter. Listen carefully and openly to what is said. A good listener is one who can appreciate how another 'sees' the world and can communicate this under-standing (empathy). Techniques that facilitate effective listening include:

  (i) making continuation responses – 'I see'. 'Go on' or 'Mm-hmm';
  (ii) reflection of feeling and content, i.e. putting into your own words what the person seems to be feeling and thinking – 'Sounds as if you've been feeling sore about the incident for some time?' Phrasing your reflection in a questioning manner allows the other the opportunity to correct any misinterpretation you may have made;
  (iii) non-verbal communication, for example looking concerned and nodding when serious issues are being discussed;
  (iv) asking open questions - 'Can you say a little more about that?' or 'What sorts of problem does this create for you?';
  (v) asking questions that directly relate to what has just been said.

- *Be reassuring in what you say and do.* A warm and friendly approach coupled with an air of quiet confidence and control, will help the other person to feel safe. People who are in tune/out of tune with each other tend to match/mismatch each other non-verbally (Morris, 1977). Therefore, one should try to match the aggressor's friendly behaviour and meet the aggressive behaviour not with anger but with concern, gradually bringing the level down to calmness.

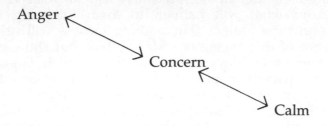

(Hall, 1988)

If you are standing, an appearance of being relaxed (and non-threatening) can be easily achieved (Picture 1). This posture has other advantages too, for example allowing you to move quickly should the need arise and offering a degree of protection should the other strike out. Note the relaxed facial expression – the eyes not staring, the brow unfurrowed and the lips parted normally. A model of calmness can be further

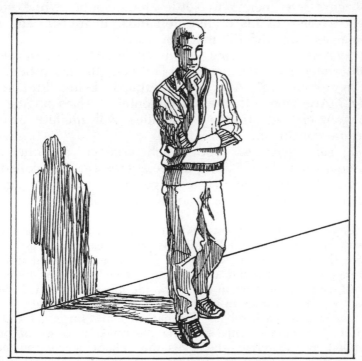

Picture 1 Safe standing position

portrayed by speaking in a clear, even tone of voice at an unhurried pace (Woodward, 1989).

People who are emotionally aroused may fear for their safety and worry about what will happen to them following the incident. Reassure the patient that nothing terrible will result as a consequence of this encounter. Make offers that show you want to consider other ways to resolve the conflict. Suggest things that the patient might do to control emotion. For example, you might say, 'Maybe it would help if we both could unwind a bit. I'm going to sit down and think for a moment about how this all started. This might help us sort this out. Why don't you try this too?' or 'Maybe it would help us both to cool off a bit if we said how we think we can end this without us both getting upset further'. Be ready with a couple of suggestions if the other person does not want to go first.

- *Avoid situations where the other person fears loss of face through backing down.* Not wanting to look like a loser turns an encounter into a fight. At all times avoid power struggles, and try to negotiate a compromise. Aim for a settlement in which both of you contribute: the aggressor may agree to think about less aggressive means to settle the dispute, while you may agree to some of his or her demands. If appropriate, remove yourselves from the influence of others.
- *Ask yourself what is going on in the immediate environment that might be prolonging the incident.* For example, are others stirring the aggressor up? Are you, perhaps, being influenced by others? Are there other environmental stresses on the patient and yourself? All these possibilities will militate against an amicable conclusion.
- *Avoid 'pat' responses.* Too much reliance on one or two techniques may be irritating to the aggressee. The skilled helper requires the ability to use a range of responses in aggressive encounters. Consider the following examples.

A 10 year old patient, on being approached by a nurse says, 'Stay away from me, you bitch!' (at this point the nurse is 6–8 feet away from the patient). Nurse replies, 'That's smart of you not to trust strangers. Never mind calling me "bitch" though, because that word could mean a lot of things beside me. Call me "G". Now pick out two chairs for us to sit in so we can learn more about whether or not to trust each other.' The patient looks surprised and meekly selects two chairs. This example illustrates a range of principles applied by the nurse: she gives the patient space; she makes an observation on what the patient's statement might mean without belittling him; she applies a limit to his behaviour with an explanation; she offers a degree of control to the client by allowing him to select the chairs; she expresses a willingness to discuss the issue further.

(Beckmann Murray and Huelskoetter, 1983)

In the next example, the incident took place on a psychiatric ward.

A man had caused so much disturbance and anxiety that police and dogs had to be brought onto the ward. The situation remained extremely tense and frightening until a nurse suggested to the patient that if he would get into bed, she would see about getting rid of all the people, the dogs and associated pressure and unpleasantness.

(Lowe, 1990)

Here the nurse offers a compromise that 'saves face' for all concerned. She also strengthens her control of the patient's behaviour – being in bed is incompatible with aggressiveness towards others. It may, in fact, further reduce his aggressiveness as he has time to cool down in a neutral environment.

• *At all times be respectful and courteous.* Be prepared to accept that the aggressor may have good reason for being angry. Do not judge until you have heard the 'full story'. As Sieff (1990) puts it when talking about the need for managers to provide good service to customers, 'Whether one is a customer along the chain of production, a customer in a shop or a customer for a service, the customer is not always right but he must not be allowed to feel when he makes a complaint that he is starting off in the wrong. On the contrary, he must be treated as though he is right . . . it is important for a customer to feel that his complaint is being properly and seriously dealt with'.

We have deliberately avoided suggestions that encourage the aggressor to engage in physical activity, such as punching a pillow or strenuous physical actions, as there is some evidence that the hoped-for cathartic effect of such behaviours, far from reducing aggression, may, in fact, have the opposite effect, i.e. increasing one's aggressive feelings. It would also appear to be the case that allowing the aggressor to overreact verbally serves to increase his or her tendency to aggress on future occasions (Aronson, 1980). One reason for these outcomes is that when we get angry we not only feel angry but also think angrily. When we vent our aggression (either physically or verbally) towards another, we may alter our perception of that person so that further acts of aggression towards that individual are likely. For example, a nurse may tell a junior colleague off in a hostile manner. She now 'feels' bad about this. To overcome her uncomfortable 'feelings', she can either convince herself that the junior was indeed at fault, thereby making it easier to be angry towards the junior on subsequent occasions, or she may apologise to the junior. For most of us the latter option is likely to be the more difficult, and it may also be less likely, as it may result in loss of face. However, it is not the case that we should not talk about our aggressive feelings. Allowing any individual to express angry feelings without overreaction, in a sympathetic environment, can reduce the likelihood of further aggression.

Talking over aims to take the heat out of the encounter and paves the way for constructive dialogue that seeks non-violent means for conflict resolution. It is an active response to encounters, based on awareness of self and other. In every encounter, we should look at the total picture before choosing our response. The comments of Dass and Gorman (1985) are relevant here:

> In skilful, helping action, when our awareness remains quiet and clear, there's breadth to our perspective. It's aerial, wide-screen, panoramic and yet able to focus quickly. With all this we are not only thinker-participants but observers of our thinking and participation as well . . . so the quiet mind makes possible an overall awareness of the total situation, including ourselves.

To help another, we have to take the reins to control our own views and opinions in order to have the time to understand how our aggressors are thinking and feeling. Politicians are well aware of the need for understanding the mentality of opponents when negotiating a settlement. Aggressive encounters should be seen as opportunities for negotiation and amicable settlement; there should not be an idea of the winner and the loser. From experience, so-called victories have only served to prolong patient resentment. Increasingly, we have come to realise that the skills required for conflict resolution are a combination of careful listening and suspended judgement, an awareness of when to be firm and when to yield a little, when to let go and when to persist, and, finally, a willingness to engage in self-exploration and a commitment to want to understand the other. These insights come from our personal experiences and, as Dass and Gorman point out:

> These insights don't come easily. It takes a great deal to detach ourselves from our vested interests and opinions long enough to take in and really feel the views of those arrayed against us . . . As fellow parents, workers, football fans – hawks and doves, we're both birds? Perhaps, but it's not always that easy in the midst of a struggle

. . . we've an obligation not to miss whatever possibilities there may be for reconciliation.

This is not to imply that we advocate that the nurse should always back down or tolerate aggression as a legitimate form of communication. Talking over is often just a first step in negotiating change. That said, talking over will sometimes not be enough or will not be appropriate to begin with. When aggressive behaviour is a serious threat to safety or property, it often has to be met with a physical response. This is discussed fully on page 79ff. However, even where restraint is necessary, we should aim for speedy resolution, with the least possible damage to the patient's self-esteem. In this way, we leave an opening for talking over at a later time. From our experience, though, in both general and pyschiatric health care settings, we believe that the majority of nurse–patient encounters will be best served by a commitment to talking over.

To increase effectiveness further, it is well worth practising a range of possible responses to the 'aggressive behaviours' that are common in the work environment. This is best done in a group context where, perhaps, each member responds in turn to a situation and a consensus is then sought as to which was the 'best' response. Reasons why some responses are better than others should be discussed.

LONG-TERM HELP TO CONTROL AGGRESSION

Talking over is intended as an immediate response to aggressive behaviours and also as a short-term strategy. In this section, we outline some longer-term measures to control anger. These are suitable for patients whose aggressive behaviour seems habitual. Feindler (1979), Feindler and Fremouw (1983), Feindler et al (1980) and Feindler et al (1984, in Goldstein and Keller, 1987) suggest a 10-week training programme. Following an introduction, participants are introduced to using a 'hassle log'. Essentially, a hassle log is a diary account of each aggressive incident experienced by the participant. Information recorded includes:

- date, time and place of the incident;
- what happened (for example, 'I was teased');
- details of the other party;
- details of the participant's response;
- outcome of the incident;
- self-evaluation of how well the participant handled the incident, together with a rating – 'burning' to 'not angry at all' – of the participant's anger.

Participants are required to bring their hassle log to each training session, and role plays are enacted based on the information in the logs. Participants are trained in five areas of arousal reduction – triggers, cues, reminders, reducers and self-evaluation – which are taught incrementally during the 10 sessions.

Triggers are the external events and internal self-statements that serve to provoke anger.

Cues refer, in this context, to the physiological experiences one has when aggressive. These experiences may be confused with other emotions such as anxiety and fear. The person is taught to recognise the feelings that are, for him or her, indicators of being aggressive, a necessary first step in making decisions to control aggression. Reflecting on the external and internal events that produce aggression and recognising when one is becoming more angry precede the next part of the anger control training package.

Reminders are taught to participants to function as counters to internal triggers. There are two main types of reminders. Generic reminders are designed to reduce anger in any situation and in response to any provocation. Examples are, 'calm down', 'keep your hat on' and 'I can cope without getting too upset'. Specific reminders are ones that have direct pertinence to that particular encounter, for example 'Perhaps he's had a difficult meeting this morning and this is his way of dealing with it' or 'I know I'm not to blame for the mistake, but right now it's best I let her have her say. There will be a better time to discuss my innocence'.

Reducers carry on from the anger reducing effect of the reminders. Participants are taught a number of ways to reduce their anger, from the relatively simple – counting backwards, deep breathing and imagining a peaceful scene – to the relatively difficult – imagining the long-term consequences of one's behaviour, for example 'I can get what I want by being violent, but I may also get sent to another institution'. Assertion techniques are also suggested as possible reducers.

The final skill taught is *self-evaluation*. Participants are taught to assess how well the preceding techniques were used, to reward themselves when the skills were used well and to self-correct when they were used poorly.

The above procedure and techniques constitute the main elements of Feindler's Anger Control Training Programme. However, use is also made of other strategies, including assertion training, problem solving training, contracting and relaxation training. In relation to the nurse–patient context, we should also consider environmental manipulation, i.e. reducing as far as possible environmental situations that may produce aggression. Of course, reducing environmental triggers has to be considered with respect to, on the one hand, helping the patient to adapt to stress in the environment and, on the other, adapting the environment to reduce the patient's stress.

In helping patients who, because of mental or intellectual impairment, might not benefit from the above programme, interventions that reward non-aggressive behaviour are recommended. These may take the form of praise, acts of friendship and more tangible reinforcers, such as trips to the cinema. As far as possible aggressive incidents should be 'played down' so that aggression is not inadvertently rewarded by giving it undue attention. Calm and relaxed periods should be strengthened by the potent reinforcers of nursing time and attention (Lyttle, 1986). The aim should be for warm and friendly relationships, based on trust and understanding. 'Blanket' ward policies to cater for all situations should be avoided. The use of patient care plans, which are regularly reviewed, will help to maintain patient individuality. The patient should be engaged in rewarding, meaningful activity. The expectation should be that all patients can contribute in some way, however small, to help raise their own self-esteem, although it should be emphasised that patients who have been in hospital for a long time may need encouragement to continue with a regular activity. Activities may include basic social skills training and projects that have a work orientation. With respect to long-stay patients suffering from schizophrenia, we have found the provision of a structured day very beneficial for most patients. We are frequently reminded by our former patients of the happy times they had when they engaged in gardening and other work-based hospital projects, yet these projects happened 10 years ago. It would appear that the patients are reflecting on a time when they felt they had a degree of self-worth and self-esteem. A structured day can be beneficial in other respects, too. If patients are left alone, their level of social withdrawal may increase. Implementing any programme of care must be consistent, as many long-stay patients have lost the ability to summon up the high level of motivation required to adapt their behaviour to frequent changes in staff expectations.

Achieving high staff enthusiasm for motivating patients in what at times will seem like an uphill battle, as patient progress may be slow and some patients will be resistive towards new interventions, calls for a high level of staff skill and commitment. It is, therefore, important that staff think carefully about how they can ensure their own continued motivation (Salmon and

Farrell, 1983). We accept, however, that the above contentions will be emotive. Some staff may feel that patients should not be actively encouraged to join an activity if they show any resistance. Our own experience suggests that staff are often polarised with regard to deciding what is best for patients. Some staff support a 'liberal' attitude, i.e. they encourage patients to be 'themselves', emphasise the need for allowing the patient to decide for himself what he wants to do and stress the importance of developing relationships. Patient aggression is seen as self-expression to be experienced and tolerated. Other staff see the need for directing and guiding patients. They emphasise routines and the use of medication to control behaviour. Aggressive incidents are seen solely in terms of patient transgression and are dealt with swiftly and 'efficiently'. Security and control are seen as priority issues at all times. We are not arguing here for either approach, as each has its own shortcomings. At worst, the permissive view may lead to tolerance and acceptance of violence, whereas the control perspective may lead to overreliance on rules, which may serve to increase the patient's sense of frustration or lead to passive acceptance. What we are suggesting is the provision of a therapeutic environment whereby liberal attitudes are tempered by the need for firm control as and when the situation arises.

Finally, careful use of medication may be effective in reducing triggers for aggression; for example the phenothiazine group of drugs can help to reduce delusional behaviour. This, in turn, can increase the accessibility of patients for therapeutic activities. A drawback is that there may be overreliance on medication, so that it may be used as a substitute for interpersonal intervention.

LIMIT SETTING

Some patients may, despite the nurse's best efforts, continue to threaten, invading his or her personal space, or damaging property. Setting limits on the patient's behaviour essentially entails informing patients calmly and directly what behaviour is and is not acceptable and calmly describing the consequences for unacceptable behaviour. Consequences may range from asking the patient to leave the ward for 20 minutes to withdrawal of certain privileges. Three principles should be borne in mind when deciding on consequences:

1. that they keep within professional acceptability;
2. that staff resources are adequate to apply them;
3. that other interventions have failed.

Once a limit is in force, the consequences must be applied immediately, otherwise the patient may manipulate staff by pointing out differences between them.

Staff cooperation is essential to ensure consistent implementation of programmes. However, some staff may be reluctant to comply with these programmes for moral and ethical reasons, whereas other staff may fear that patients will react aggressively towards them and a few staff may apply the limit so assiduously that they could be accused of being punitive towards the patient. It is, therefore, imperative that all programmes are carefully monitored and that staff and patient views are regularly sought. Any disagreements between staff must be confined to staff meetings and not 'spill over' to the patient. Limit setting is rarely an end in itself, rather a means to an end. It offers interim control of a patient's aggressive behaviour until other interventions can be tried. As far as possible, the patient should be involved in discussions about what the consequences should be, otherwise his or her sense of powerlessness may serve to increase the isolation and alienation from staff. In fact, these discussions should be seen as a 'back door' entry to longer-term anger control training programmes, as the patient is encouraged to think about alternatives to his or her continuing aggression.

RESPONDING TO EMERGENCIES

As each situation is unique, the best technique in the most ideal circumstances may not be enough to contain an incident. Some staff may think they have failed if they cannot contain a situation themselves, and a feeling of 'losing one's grip' on the situation may precipitate hasty or ill thought out actions. Knowing when to seek help should be seen as an extension of the nurse's aggression management skills, not as an end to them. This section focuses on what might be done in situations which appear to be getting out of hand and where help is needed. Essentially, the nurse has two choices: getting out and getting help.

'Getting out' refers to the ways in which a nurse may withdraw from a situation. It is usually a preliminary to getting help, whereby the support of others is sought. Sometimes, during an incident, it is sensible to position oneself safely while working out the next move. Some experienced staff do this automatically, for example, keeping a good arm's distance away from the other person, subtly positioning themselves behind a barrier (such as a table) and keeping exits within sight and reach. A retreat from the situation might be achieved by making a plausible excuse or simply saying, 'I'm going to go now'.

Try this exercise on getting help.

ACTIVITY 7

How might help be obtained in an emergency in your work setting?

Now see the discussion below.

Discussion

There are usually several options in an emergency, and the choice should be made in light of a quick assessment of the situation.

In some circumstances it may be expedient to *run* for help, or, alternatively, you could *send someone* else (a colleague or a patient, for example) for help. *Shouting* may be appropriate, and in some situations it may be sensible to lock yourself in a room and call for help from an open window.

Some areas have a 'panic button': perhaps linking the bedrooms, offices/consulting rooms, with the main ward. A bleep system is often also used in emergencies.

The *fire alarm* may be used if other means of summoning assistance are not to hand, and in some settings *personal alarms* are appropriate.

In institutional settings, one should not forget the *telephone*, and one should be aware of the number to call as it can vary from hospital to hospital. Some hospitals also have special call-up numbers for an emergency. These need to be pointed out to bank staff, in particular, for example, when handing the ward over to one who is not familiar with local customs. Dialling 999 on a *public phone* might be another course of action. Finally *car phones* should be considered for some community workers.

Having a readily available, easy-to-use means of summoning assistance is important, but it should not be seen as a substitute for adequate staffing levels and proper training. Pressing a call button too early may only serve to escalate an attack. If staff often need to press a 'panic button', the reason for this needs investigation. For example, are the staffing resources adequate, does the staff member lack the appropriate skills, does the physical environment need to be changed so that staff are not so vulnerable? The other side of the coin is that anyone receiving a distress call should react promptly.

Where departments have reciprocal arrangements to help one another, it should be clear among the staff who will attend emergencies. This might need deciding daily, depending on circumstances, which will prevent time being wasted on deciding who should go when the time arises.

All wards should have an agreed procedure on handling incidents of aggression. Staff should know how help is obtained on their unit, and it should be made clear who is responsible for decision making in crisis situations and the importance of a team approach.

WHEN RESTRAINT IS REQUIRED

Restraint may be necessary for the following reasons (Department of Health, 1990a page 74):

- Physical assault.
- Destructive behaviour.
- Non-compliance with treatment.
- Self-harm or risk of physical injury by accident.
- Overactivity likely to result in exhaustion.

Nobody can prescribe when and when not to restrain. In each situation, one has to weigh up the pros and cons of intervening. It might be preferable to have a few chairs smashed than risk injury to oneself or others, but if it looks as if all the furniture is going to be damaged, one might decide that an intervention is justified. Although restraint is not the most enjoyable part of nurses' work, it is nevertheless an aspect of care that requires the same degree of attention as other care practices. It is important to remember that the other person has a right to professional care even when he or she is aggressive, so the minimum amount of force should be used in restraint. You are not expected to restrain single-handedly, as you can put yourself and the other at risk of being injured. In fact, the best policy is not to restrain on your own unless it is absolutely unavoidable. Remember that restraint should only be used as a means of control when other non-physical attempts have failed. Some departments may have a policy that, whenever possible, nursing staff do not restrain, this being left to other non-nursing personnel, such as security staff or the police.

GUIDELINES FOR PHYSICAL RESTRAINT

The effect of physical restraint is usually to curtail a patient's movement for a short period of time. An elderly confused patient, for example, may only need to be approached from behind and turned by the shoulders to face in the direction of a safer environment. However, sometimes, where serious violence or self-harm seems imminent, it may be appropriate for the patient to be temporarily immobilised. The effects of this are to prompt the patient to reconsider his or her actions and to avert harm. This kind of restraint requires practical skill and understanding, and it is on this that we focus in this section of the book.

Where staff may be called from another area, they invariably arrive at the scene without knowledge of the type of situation needing help. The emergency call invariably comes *after* an incident involving aggression, and its aim is to protect staff and patients from further harm. Here, the visiting staff members need to assemble and receive a briefing from the ward staff, to ensure a team response. Occasionally, however, staff will arrive to find an incident in progress and must decide whether or not to intervene immediately. Normally, it is best for an individual not to tackle the aggressor alone, but where another person is obviously being harmed, 'first aid' is required. Verbal restraint should be considered first; a command to refrain or desist may suffice for some individuals. Otherwise, the aggressor could be pushed away or some other means tried of enabling the victim to escape (e.g. distraction or the breakaway techniques outlined in Chapter 8). Once the action is interrupted, many patients accept that as an end to the message being communicated. If it seems vital to intervene physically on your own (e.g. to preserve life), the chances of succeeding must be weighed up against the possibility and effect of injury. Aggression resulting in serious injury, as it occasionally does, can rarely be affected by the intervention of one person. Here, one's priority should be to preserve oneself and muster support as quickly as possible.

Where physical restraint is unavoidable, the following points are seen as good practice:

- Identify one nurse to be in charge of the restraint, and ensure that everyone knows who it is who will guide them. The person appointed to coordinate may be the patient's nurse (key-worker or primary nurse) and should attempt to calm the patient through the use of interpersonal skills.
- Assess the situation. While help is gathering, the nurse who has assumed responsibility should establish that the environment is a safe one in which to carry out the restraint. He or she should make a visual check of the patient for weapons.

Furniture and artefacts that could cause injury or themselves be damaged should be removed if possible, and onlookers should be shepherded away.

- Assemble an adequate number of staff. Premeditated restraint on someone known to be resistive should never be attempted with fewer than five staff, not including anyone, for example, who might be needed to administer a drug. At this stage, verbal restraint should be tried again, because a few firm words by the nurse coordinating, together with a show of strength, may be enough to defuse the situation. The Code of Practice (Department of Health, 1990a) states that staff should attempt to get the patient's agreement to stop before using restraint, explaining the consequences where possible. Furthermore, anyone not involved should be asked to leave.

- Observe restraint ethics. The reason why restraint is safe and effective can be attributed to the tendency of staff to maintain certain standards:

  (i) Acknowledge your own level of preparedness for restraining patients. Professional behaviour requires that the nurse can identify his or her shortcomings and, ideally, take steps to obtain, develop or update the necessary skills before they are needed. Also, satisfy yourself about the competence of colleagues. New and inexperienced staff may think that they understand their role, but the actual instance of aggression is not the time to find out otherwise.

  (ii) Be committed to the restraint. The nurse who is uncertain of his or her ability or desire to participate may put everyone at risk. Half-hearted attempts can easily result in unnecessary harm. If you are uncertain about intervening, let the coordinating nurse know as early as possible.

  (iii) Establish the aim of the restraint in each case. The immediate aim will normally be obvious, but if any treatment is to be given compulsorily while the patient is immobilised, the coordinating nurse should ensure that he or she can justify its use. Restraint must be lawful.

  (iv) Prepare yourself for physical contact. Remove any dangerous items which may be on your person. Pens, watches, spectacles, dangling earrings and certain other items could injure staff or patient or be damaged. Ties and scarves may choke if pulled by the patient in a struggle.

  (v) Apply force safely when restraining. Using five nurses enables one to restrain each limb while the fifth takes responsibility for the head. It is this nurse who should

continue talking to the patient to explain what is going on
and to monitor the patient's response to the restraint. He
or she should protect the head and neck from possible
injury and gauge when it is safe to discontinue the
restraint. The other nurses should hold the limbs near the
major joints (upper arms and thighs) as this minimises the
lever effect. Excessive twisting or bending of the limbs
should be avoided as fractures or dislocation may result.
If biting is attempted, the patient's hair can be held firmly.
Some patients continue to threaten harm after they have
been immobilised, and where this occurs, it can be safer
to turn them into the prone position. Remember, if
applicable, to unfasten the patient's trousers beforehand
when medication is likely to be required, and inform the
patient of your intentions.

(vi) Any form of restraint should be time-limited and must
never be used continuously for longer than 8 hours. For
periods of restraint in excess of 1 hour, review times must
be specified in advance.

• Make provisions for care after the restraint. A period of
seclusion is often prescribed following an incident which
requires the use of restraint. This may require a single room to
be prepared, perhaps with a mattress on the floor, and the re-
deployment of staff. While the restrainers are waiting for the
patient to calm down, sedation can be considered, and if
appropriate, this can be made ready and given at this time.
Note that sedation should be *offered* in the first place.

In the course of the restraint an important principle of control
involves limiting the extent to which the patient can use the lever
action of the arms and legs; by holding the limbs near to the
major joints it is possible to reduce the amount of force they can
exert. The following two situations illustrate this point.

Situation 1. A confused elderly patient insists on 'going home',
and persuading him to return to the ward has little effect. In this
situation two people may be enough to restrain safely and with
dignity.

Note that the elbow and shoulder joints permit powerful
leverage action. The nurses can control the movement in these
two joints by linking each arm, as shown in picture 2, and
holding the patient's wrists, as in picture 3. As far as possible, a
relaxed but alert approach should be adopted, the nurse talking
to the patient to allay his anxiety and encourage compliance.

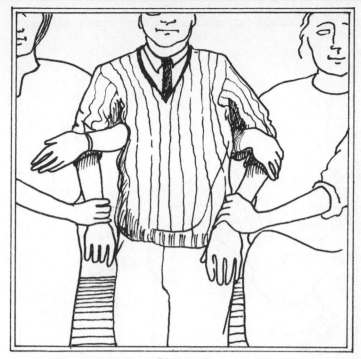

Picture 2

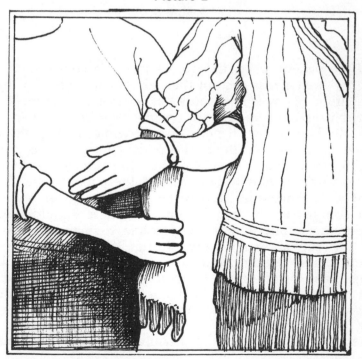

Picture 3

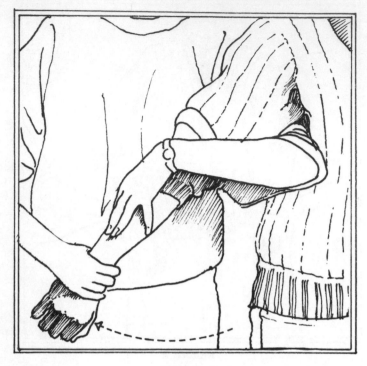

Picture 4

Should the patient resist, the nurses can gain control by bringing one of his arms across each of their abdomens, while at the same time rotating his wrists inwards, as shown in picture 4. If the patient refuses to move forward despite requests to do so, motion can usually be resumed if both nurses, while holding the patient as shown in picture 4, 'push' the patient forwards, as shown in picture 5. Note that, to achieve this, the nurses are bending a little so as to put their weight behind the patient's shoulders.

Situation 2. Sometimes it may be necessary to immobilise the patient completely. In these situations, there should ideally be five restrainers, but it may be possible to manage with fewer where the patient is not very strong. When three nurses are involved in the restraint, one nurse can immobilise the legs by keeping them together and by putting her weight on the lower part of the limbs, as shown in picture 6. The nurses holding the patient's arms achieve maximum control by holding them firmly in the position shown in picture 7. This manœuvre is not designed to hurt the patient. Normally, the restrainer should aim

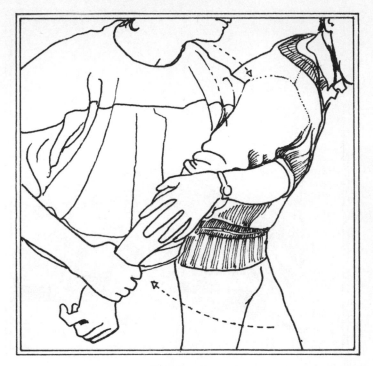

Picture 5

to hold in a 'relaxed' but vigilant manner; only if the patient struggles is there a need to apply much force.

Finally, note that the aggressor is held in a prone position. If he tries to damage himself by banging his head against the ground, one of the nurses holding an arm controls his head movements by getting into the position shown in picture 8. (The patient should, of course, never be held around the neck.) This nurse should take responsibility for monitoring the patient's airway.

When the aggressor is large relative to the size of the restrainers, more help will be required, but the principle, i.e. *immobilisation depends on the control of levers*, remains the same.

Restraint is not a measure to be carried out without appreciating the need to continue supporting the patient psychologically. On its own, restraint may simply produce frustration and bitterness, so throughout the restraint one nurse should continue to talk to the patient. This nurse should explain what is happening and

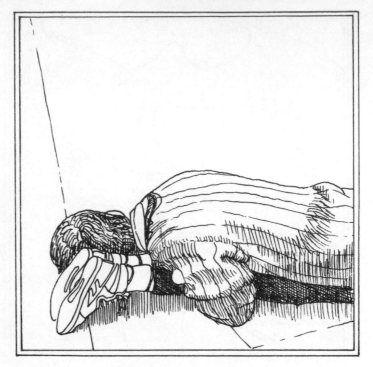

Picture 6 Leg restraint

what is intended, and should adopt a calming, but firm, tone of voice, indicating that the nurses are in control and are not going to allow anyone to be harmed. Engaging the patient in conversation will also distract his or her attention and reduce attempts to harm the restrainers. A speedy end to the ordeal should be aimed for. The patient's cooperation should be sought without recourse to threats of the consequences of continuing disturbed behaviour. Often when calm again, the patient will agree that the condition warrants them taking a tranquillising drug and spending a period in a quiet environment. The nurses will offer to release their grip when the patient can agree not to hit out, but the release should be carried out carefully, with the nurses ready to take control again if required. Kaplan and Wheeler (1983) suggest that after an aggressive incident arousal levels remain high for up to 90 minutes. Therefore, staff should be particularly careful to avoid situations that might incite a recurrence of the aggression, hence the value of diminishing the stimulation in the environment.

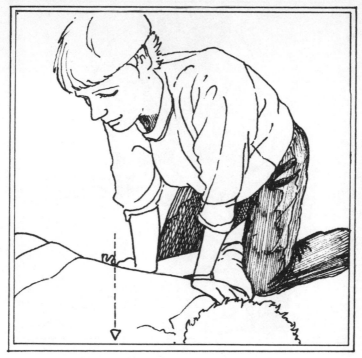

Picture 7   Downward force on joints

BYSTANDERS

Aggression often occurs in the presence of people who have no real involvement with the incident. Patients and relatives may be at the scene, as may staff who work elsewhere in the hospital, and all these can compound the risk of someone getting hurt. There are many advantages in, where possible, preventing aggression from taking place in front of bystanders, who should normally be ushered away as quietly as possible. Apart from the danger to themselves, some have been known to want to pitch in to help either the nurses or the patient! It is also possible that having an audience may serve to prolong an incident, as the aggressor feels that backing down would mean public humiliation.

However, if a nurse were facing a difficult situation with no staff support on hand, it would be expedient to send a bystander for help. Note, though, that a group of people can produce a divided responsibility in such circumstances. In the notorious

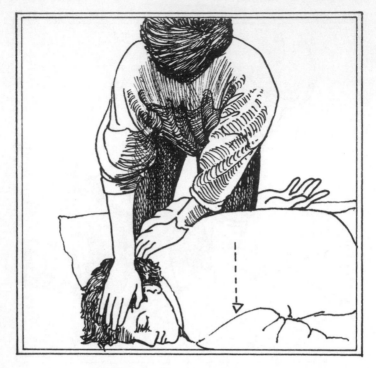

Picture 8   Head in safe position

Kitty Genovese murder case (Rosenthal, 1964), about 40 people heard the victim screaming for half an hour before she died. Not one of them called the police, apparently because each thought that someone else might do it. If a number of people stand around looking to each other for reference points to the correct behaviour for the circumstances, all of them delude themselves that it is acceptable to do nothing. It seems that the presence of others tends to define the situation as a non-emergency, while diffusing the responsibility for acting (Atkinson et al., 1990). The lesson for us here is that one bystander should be named and specifically instructed in how to get help.

Finally, witnesses to aggression may well find the experience very frightening; the need to offer them further support is explored on page 126.

MECHANICAL RESTRAINT

'Mechanical restraint' defines the curtailing of a patient's freedom of movement by means of a mechanical device, and is a form of physical restraint. Numerous examples of mechanical restraint exist, including cotsides, harnesses and barrier chairs. It should be stressed that an arrangement of furniture that impedes movement may also be viewed as mechanical restraint.

Although most of these devices have been available for many years as aids to the management of aggression, their general use is now widely frowned upon within the caring professions. Staff shortages can seduce any of us into thinking that using a mechanical restrainer will save nursing time. But, as well as the infringement of the patient's liberty that they cause, many have been found to be dangerous. A common problem is that the application of one of these devices, for example a barrier chair, can lead the nurse to believe that a patient is immobile and, therefore, 'safe' from harm. However, the patient may continue his or her efforts to be free, the behaviour that probably caused the nurse to instigate sanctions in the first place. This nurse then fails properly to observe what is happening and is unaware of the effect on the patient. Any physical injury will be discovered later, but the emotional trauma may never be fully appreciated. Confused patients can easily misinterpret the purpose of restraining devices (as can relatives), and when this is likely, they should not be used. Mechanical restraint must not be used as an alternative to constant observation, and, therefore, rather than being an aid to patient care, it may only be safe when adequate staff are available.

It has been suggested (Royal College of Nursing, 1987) that it may be acceptable in some situations to use mechanical restraint with the confused elderly, providing that elementary precautions are observed. These precautions are described elsewhere in this book but, broadly, they include using restraint as a last resort, for a limited period of time, and ensuring that the reasons for its use have been documented. This guide also offers useful information on alternatives to mechanical restraint, i.e. reorientation and creating a more suitable environment.

The recommendation from the Confederation of Health Service Employees (1977), however, is that no mechanical restraint should be used in any circumstances whatsoever. Where it is used by staff without the patient's consent, and especially if the device has not been authorised by the health authority, it may well amount to an assault. Also, because staff are not constantly involved, mechanical restraint may tend to be left in place for a period longer than may be reasonable in the circumstances – an example of false imprisonment. Clearly, here is another issue that nurses should discuss widely and seek clarification of the legal implications for their particular practice.

CHEMICAL RESTRAINT

Although drugs are widely prescribed for aggression, claims that they can be used to *treat* aggressive behaviour are difficult to substantiate. It is probably more accurate to argue that drugs treat the psychiatric problems associated with aggression, rather than aggression itself. It is important to recognise this because it forces us to question the practice of the prolonged routine use of certain drugs in patients who are inclined to be aggressive. Rather than having a therapeutic effect, this practice could be seen more as restraint. Furthermore, this can produce the worst kind of restraint – without any time limit and without the necessary psychological support for the patient. In short, if it can be shown that the drug regime used amounts to chemical restraint, the practice may be unlawful, especially perhaps where informal patients are concerned or where the drugs must be administered by force.

The Code of Practice (Department of Health, 1990a) requires nurses to debate the purpose of sedative drugs when they are in long-term use. The UKCC Code of Conduct (1984) could be seen as supporting this idea through its concern with the role of the nurse as the patient's advocate. People with learning difficulties or with so-called burnt-out schizophrenia, and even children, may need special representation. What is asked is that where patients are subject to prolonged sedative drug therapy, there should be regular discussion and review for each individual concerned. Nurses should reassess these patients frequently and consider alternatives to drugs. The Code of Practice also emphasises that drug therapy should not be used as an alternative to adequate staffing.

In the acute general setting, similar caution should be exercised, even though this kind of nursing may not be thought of as being governed by mental health legislation. It is not uncommon to use tranquillisers, especially where aggression accompanies confusion. The intravenous administration of chlormethiazole (Heminevrin), for example, produces extremely effective sedation, but staff should be alert that this type of chemical restraint is not abused simply because patients who can be aggressive are not pleasant people to nurse. Neither should this use of drugs be accepted instead of adequate staffing levels necessary for intensive nursing ('specialling').

Further problems could arise if nurses try to avoid disturbing the aggressive patient once the drugs have taken effect – an especially easy option on any busy ward. Letting 'sleeping dogs lie' can result in dehydration, pressure sores or incontinence. Clearly, many elements of the common law could be relevant here, and professional practice should result in a nurse having a lawful justification for everything he or she does. One aspect of this is that even where sedation is unavoidable, it will at least be accompanied by evidence that its use was agreed upon by the team, ideally in consultation with the relatives, that it was short term and that a review time was set up at the outset.

INFECTION CONTROL

It is important that infection control be considered here. The need for restraint may be prompted by self-injurious behaviour, or it may *cause* injury to the patient, resulting in blood loss. Specific testing (for example for human immuno-deficiency virus; HIV) is not usually carried out, and the recommendation (Royal College of Nursing, 1985) is that consequently, every precaution should be taken in all cases.

The risk of HIV being transmitted during a violent incident is small. The only likely means is by blood from an infected individual contaminating an open wound, bite or scratch. However, the correct first aid should be administered if this occurs, and blood spillages should also be properly dealt with to protect others.

No less important in these circumstances is the risk of contracting other blood-borne viruses, such as hepatitis B. Here, spitting may also put staff in danger, and, in the event of this, staff should take action in accordance with their local infection control policy. Staff health departments should be consulted for immunisation advice. For further information and advice see *Guidance for Clinical Health Care Workers: Protection Against Infection with HIV and Hepatitis Viruses* (Department of Health, 1990b).

END THOUGHTS

Measures to avoid an immediate recurrence of the incident should be implemented. Sometimes the actions required are obvious, for example when there is a policy already drawn up for such an

Table 2 Seclusion versus time out

	Seclusion	Time out
Length of confinement	Arbitrary time period; may be hours or days	Set time period. Rarely more than a few hours, more often a few minutes
Type of confinement	Secure or locked environment away from other patients	Restricted to own bedroom or may be asked to go off the ward
Reason for intervention	Serious incidents involving threat to self or others. Damage to property	'Minor' incidents, e.g. foul language
Patient consent	Not always given	Normally given
Relationship to anger control programmes	May or may not be a planned intervention	Part of a carefully planned programme
Rationale	Protection of patient, staff or property. Reduction of stimulation until patient gains self-control	Removal from positive reinforcement; e.g. bad language may be followed by 10 minutes in a room
Who decides	* Unless patient's doctor is actually present, nurse should decide	Usually a joint decision by all staff and patient

* Often the only personnel immediately available during an emergency situation are nursing staff. When this happens, the decision to seclude must rest with the nurse. Of course, even when a decision to seclude is 'prescribed' by the doctor, nurses must satisfy themselves that they are acting lawfully (see pages 115–20).

occurrence. When no policy exists, the person in charge will have to decide on interim measures until such time as a more detailed discussion can take place. The decision of what action to take should be based on a consideration of what is safest for all concerned and what is reasonable in the circumstances. Interim measures might include:

• keeping the person under constant observation;
• restricting the person to a room;
• asking the aggressor to leave;
• calling the police.

Restraint, whether it be physical control, as outlined above, or confinement of the patient to a secure environment, places great responsibility on the nursing staff and is not a duty to be undertaken lightly. Depriving someone of liberty must only be a last resort to save the patient from harming self or others, or to prevent damage to property. If restraint proves not to be a last resort measure, there may be a legal case to answer, so nurses have to balance the risk inherent in allowing potentially aggressive patients reasonable freedoms against the nurses' duty to care. Normally, this is accomplished most professionally.

SECLUSION

Sometimes staff use the word 'seclusion' synonymously with the words 'time out', but it is better to see these terms as lying on opposite ends of the limit setting continuum. Basically, the differences can be summed up as in Table 2.

Gibson (1989) describes the typical seclusion room as 'having no furnishings, except a mattress on the floor; walls are plain and solid. The lighting is controlled from outside the room and windows and heater are situated high on the wall out of reach. The door of the seclusion room can only be opened/locked from the outside and usually has an observation window.' It could be argued that such stark environments are rarely necessary for more than short periods of time. Incarcerating patients in bare environments is only justified when furnishings and other equipment might be used by the patient to damage him or herself or staff. Ideally, the secure environment is a self-contained unit, comprising a seclusion room, adjacent bathroom and recreational area, separated from the main ward by an anteroom. There should also be a system for summoning extra staff.

Seclusion should be seen as a therapeutic intervention rather than simply as social isolation. Baradell (1985) suggests that the seclusion experience can be thought of as consisting of three phases. The *initiation* phase begins when the decision is made to seclude a patient. The goals here are to orientate the patient to the reality of being secluded, the reduction of sensory input and the implementation of a plan of care to meet the patient's emotional and physical needs. The *reintegration* phase helps the patient to regain control over his or her thinking, feeling and behaviour and provides a moderate level of sensory input. The *reincorporation* phase plans the gradual assimilation of the patient back into the wider community. This phase is likely to be an anxious one for patient, staff and other residents. The patient may feel embarrassed and frightened, staff may be uncertain when to relinquish control and other residents may fear for their safety. Regular staff/patient meetings will help to air residents' fears and provide an opportunity for reassurance.

The following safeguards are offered by the Royal College of Nursing (1979) for the seclusion of patients:

- Whenever possible, the likely need for seclusion should be predicted.
- The duty medical officer and the duty senior nurse should be told as soon as possible, and they are expected to attend at the first opportunity.
- Seclusion should take place in an environment that is secure and where the patient cannot accidentally or intentionally harm him or herself.
- Observation should take place every 15 minutes; a full nursing review should occur not less than once every 2 hours. A secondary review should take place not less than every 4 hours, and will require the presence of a medical officer.
- When seclusion is for more than 8 hours or for more than 12 hours intermittently over a period of 48 hours, a further review procedure should be instituted.
- For prolonged seclusion, it is important that there is independence of reviewers, which may entail the presence of one of the hospital managers. Any need to prolong seclusion should also require that the patient be subject to a compulsory detention order.
- Proper records must be kept, both in the patient's notes and in a 'ward seclusion book'.
- All patients coming into a psychiatric hospital should receive an admission booklet, which explains the occasional need to segregate individual patients.
- Relatives should be kept personally informed when seclusion has been considered necessary.

NURSING THE PATIENT IN A QUIET ROOM

Sometimes patients are moved to a quiet room when they are noisy or cause disturbance to others or when a 'special eye' is being kept on the patient. The room is not locked, and patients either agree to the measure or at least do not offer resistance to being moved. If they did, this would, in effect, be seclusion and would, therefore, have to be prescribed by a doctor. The patient may be nursed in the quiet room for 24 hours or longer, or for much shorter periods of time. Nursing patients in a quiet room also requires regular careful evaluation, as it can sometimes have unsatisfactory consequences.

It is our experience of the general setting at night that elderly patients are sometimes moved from the open ward to a single room, or even put into the clinical room, when they become restless and disturbing to other patients. Often, though, these patients become even more confused when moved, probably as a result of increased disorientation brought about by the unfamiliar surroundings. As far as possible, one should try to anticipate patients' needs early to avoid unnecessary moves, looking for early warning signs that the patient is growing restless and becoming confused. It is at this stage that the nurse can take action. If it appears that the patient is disorientated, the nurse can sit with the patient and tactfully explain who he or she is and where the patient is. Calmly reassuring the patient of his or her whereabouts and taking time to listen will help to settle the patient. When the patient's words do not make sense, the nurse should *listen to the mood* (Stedeford, 1983). The author recalls the incessant cries of a 90-year-old lady, 'When is my mummy coming?', which appeared to be her way of communicating profound loneliness and fear. Being nearby and communicating friendliness were of greater comfort to this patient than any attempts to reorientate her to the reality of her situation. Other actions might include offering patients their favourite night-time drinks and attending to their basic needs: patients might grow restless if they are wet or feel the need to go to the toilet. If patients appear to be misinterpreting objects in their immediate environment, increasing the level of lighting around their beds might help. As far as possible, the patients' relatives should be involved in settling these patients at night, as having a familiar face may help to reduce their confusion. At any rate, relatives should know of the nurses' actions so that they do not misinterpret them. Careful consideration of night-time medication may also be an option. If, despite all efforts, the patient continues to be restless at night moving him or her to the side room earlier rather than later in the evening may be considered, so that he or she may have time to get used to the new surroundings.

Finally, all occasions involving seclusion and nursing in a quiet room must be documented and the safeguards outlined above adhered to. Nurses must constantly review their practice so that these occasions do not become the easy option; nurses should always be seen to be acting in the patient's best interest.

Try this exercise.

ACTIVITY 8

In what circumstances would you not be willing to restrain?
Now see the discussion below.

Discussion
Restraint in the following encounters is best left to skilled personnel, for example the police and specially trained staff:

- aggressive encounters that involve the use of a weapon, for example a knife, a broken bottle and sometimes even dogs, may be used to intimidate or threaten (see the discussion on page 112);
- situations in which you are outnumbered or the aggressor is large;
- situations in which the available staff are not properly trained for intervention.

In any situation where restraint is thought necessary, the chances of success should outweigh the chances of failure.

Further Reading

Argyle M (1988) *Bodily Communication,* 2nd edn. London: Methuen. (A good introduction to most aspects of non-verbal behaviour.)

Holden U P and Woods R T (1988) *Reality Orientation.* London: Churchill Livingstone. (A comprehensive guide to the major issues relating to RO.)

Nelson-Jones R (1988) *Practical Counselling and Helping Skills,* 2nd edn. London: Cassell. (A good introduction to communication skills in a variety of contexts.)

Royal College of Nursing (1987) *Focus on Restraint.* London: RCN. (Detailed information on the use of restraint in the care of elderly people, both in hospital and in the community.)

Royal College of Nursing Labour Relations and Legal Department (1984) *Violence – Policy Guidlines no. 17.* London: RCN. (Brief but helpful advice that must be applied at ward level.)

Smith L (1978) Limit setting. *Nursing Times,* **74** (26): 1074–5. (Describes how limit setting can be used with patients whom nurses find difficult to manage.)

7
Breakaway Techniques

Key Points

- If violence occurs when there is nobody else around, breakaway techniques can be used to permit escape.

- Breakaway techniques must be practised with suitable supervision before attempting to use them, otherwise they may be used unsuccessfully or even unnecessarily.

- The legal and professional acceptability of breakaway techniques should be considered before they are widely adopted.

- If threatened with a weapon, personal safety comes first.

WHEN VIOLENCE OCCURS AND THERE IS NO ONE ABOUT EXCEPT YOU

It is conceivable that interpersonal skills may not always serve to guarantee one's personal safety in the face of aggression. An attack could happen unexpectedly or when help is not readily available, and in this kind of situation, it may be desirable to have recourse to measures that would fend off an attacker and provide time for help to arrive. The aim of breakaway techniques, then, is primarily to *escape*, using the minimum force necessary. The brief descriptions given here are by way of an introduction only. The authors do not recommend that these techniques be tried without prior practice under skilled supervision.

Note that it is wise to view the usefulness of teaching breakaway techniques with caution. There is always a danger that they will be used unnecessarily; for example, someone may take hold of you suddenly with no further intention of causing harm, and your release can be achieved by appealing to be let go. Furthermore, there is no guarantee that your efforts will actually be successful. Clearly, in judging the situation, the nurse must

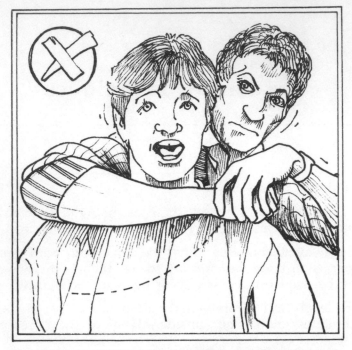

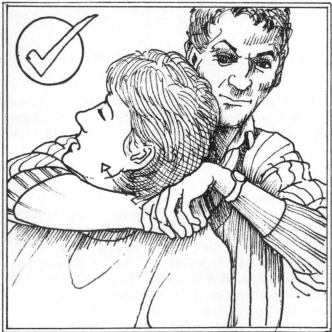

Picture 9 '. . . Maintain your airway'

decide between possibly putting him or herself in danger and completely overreacting. It is the potential for overreaction that concerns the critics of teaching breakaway techniques. The reader's attention is drawn to Chapter 8, 'The Legal Position', which discusses the scope in law for nurses to employ self-defence. This section on breakaway techniques should certainly not be seen as a first course in the martial arts.

Maintain Your Airway

Always try to avoid a situation in which someone can put pressure on your airway. Move your head so that your Adam's apple is facing towards the attacker's elbow (picture 9). Only now should you consider further escape options.

Finger Grab and Bend

The chance of being strangled may justify this manœuvre. Grab and bend back the attacker's fingers (picture 10); any fingers will do. It is possible that you may break them, but this may be your only option if you feel in serious danger.

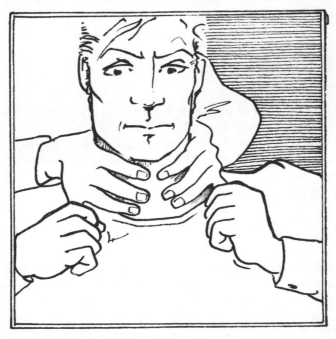

Picture 10   Finger grab and bend

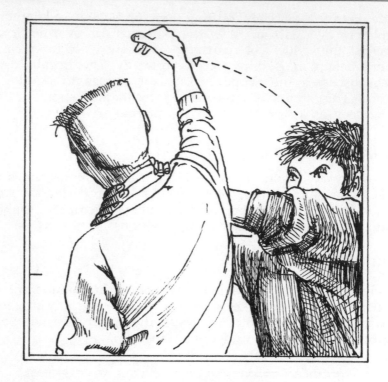

Picture 11   Bowling manœuvre

Bowling Manœuvre

Move your right leg slightly backwards so that you are positioned to move quickly to your left. Now raise your right arm and shoulder as if you were overarm bowling (picture 11). Your arm and your body should move together and then move away smartly at the point of disengagement (Woodward, 1989). For such a simple technique, this is very effective.

Holding On

If your hair is pulled, press the attacker's hands down so as to minimise the effect of the pull (picture 12). At the same time, rush towards your attacker so as to throw him or her off balance. A loud shout as you do this may increase the surprise and distraction element of the manœuvre. This approach can also be used if your necktie or scarf is pulled.

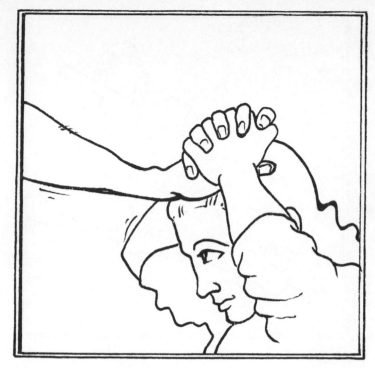

Picture 12   Holding on

Horseshoe Grip Break

Think of the attacker's hand as forming a horseshoe shape around your wrist. Break the grip by snapping through the weakest point of the grip: down and away (pictures 13 and 14). It is very important to move your body in the direction of your 'snap'; by bringing your body weight behind your snap, it will provide you with sufficient force to break your attacker's grip (Woodward, 1989).

Two-handed Grab Break

If you are grabbed so that your hand is facing downwards, break your attacker's grip by bringing your arm up and smartly away with the aid of your free hand, as shown (pictures 15 and 16).

If your arm is facing upwards when grabbed, move it downwards, again with the aid of your free hand (Woodward, 1989) (pictures 17 and 18).

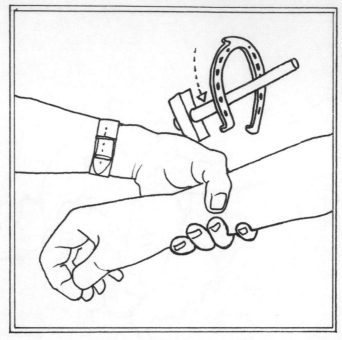

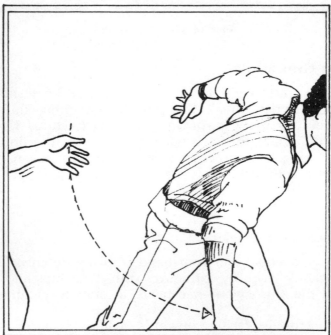

Pictures 13 & 14   'Go for the horseshoe . . .'

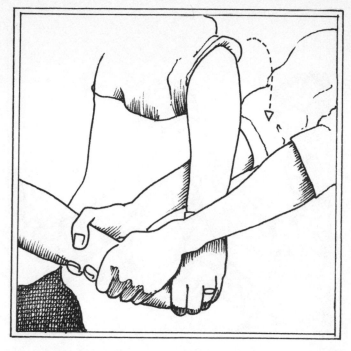

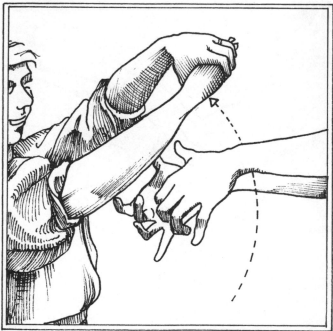

Pictures 15 & 16 Two-handed grab break (arm facing downwards)

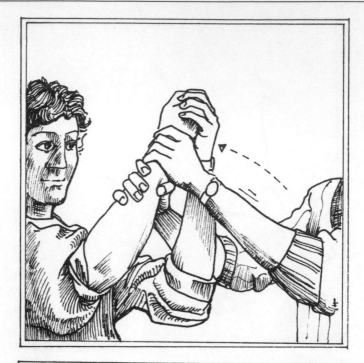

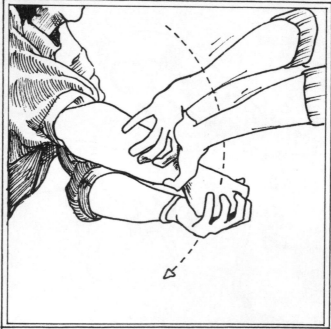

Pictures 17 & 18   Two-handed grab break (arm facing upwards)

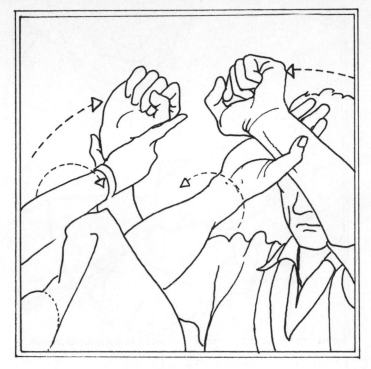

Picture 19   Two-handed roll-up

Two-hand Roll-up

If both wrists are grabbed, quickly move your wrists outwards and upwards (picture 19). Twist your wrists inwards as you do this so that the attacker will have difficulty holding onto you (Woodward, 1989).

Phoenix Fist-to-Hand

Strike hard with a hammer action on the back of the attacker's hand (picture 20). 'Scraping' down the attacker's shin with the heel of your shoe can be a useful addition to this manœuvre.

Triceps Pinch

Pinch and twist the skin on the attacker's arms (picture 21). The effect on the skin is far more painful than that on muscle, so try not to grasp muscle.

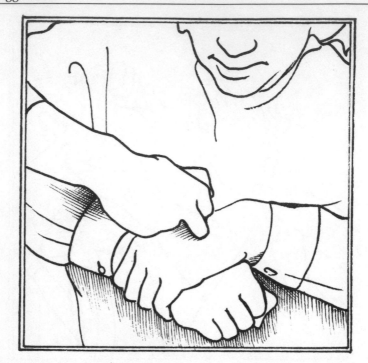

Picture 20 Phoenix fist to hand

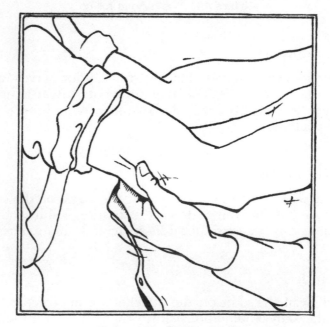

Picture 21 Triceps pinch

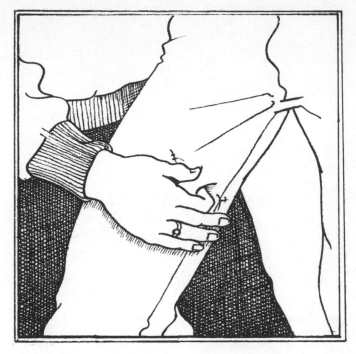

Picture 22 Thigh pinch

Thigh Pinch

Pinch and twist the skin on the attacker's inner thigh (picture 22).
This is an effective escape technique and can be used in a variety
of situations. One disadvantage is that it may not be possible
when the attacker is wearing tight jeans.

Knuckle to Sternum

Apply pressure to the attacker's sternum; push hard and twist
(picture 23). Do not use a stabbing action. You can move forward
a little as you push the attacker off. This manœuvre is possible
in a number of situations, e.g. when someone tries to 'crowd you
out' or when grabbed from the front. However, this, and some
of the other manœuvres above, rely on pain for their effectiveness. The authors advise inflicting pain only as a last resort,
because pain may go unnoticed when one is aroused and the
aggressor may not respond as desired.

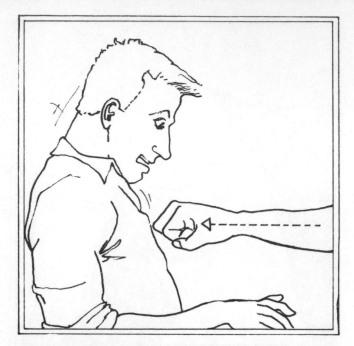

Picture 23   Knuckle to sternum

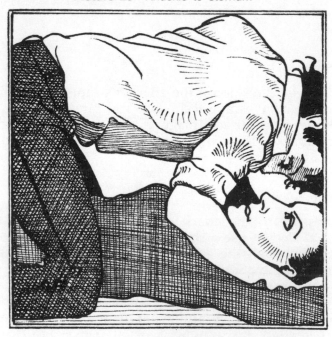

Picture 24   Stay calm and talk

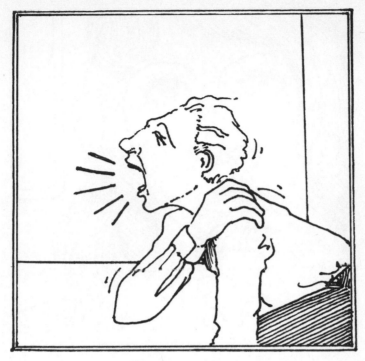

Picture 25   Feigning

Stay Calm and Talk

In situations in which both the nurse and the aggressor are immobilised and actual violence has ceased (at least for the moment), it may be worthwhile to try to talk with the attacker (picture 24). If the attacker is not harming you, there may be little need to try to escape.

Feigning

Sometimes feigning (by word and deed) the amount of damage done may cause the attacker to stop (picture 25). Even an attacker can empathise with someone who appears mortally hurt.

Behave Disgustingly

The aim here is to 'put off' the intending attacker, and it is a possibility in some instances (picture 26). You might, for example, pick your nose, spit or engage in other antisocial behaviour.

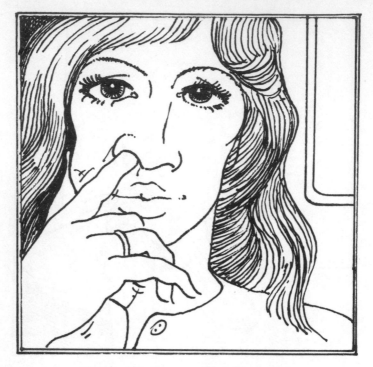

Picture 26 Do something disgusting

If the motive for the attack is remotely sexual, behaving disgustingly can serve to 'turn off' the offender.

Do Something Surprising

Do something that the intending attacker may find distracting and/or even amusing; it need not even be something novel (picture 27). Telling your attacker that you are just going to tie up your shoelace may be enough to break the tenseness of the situation and allow you to begin to take control through verbal means (Woodward, 1989).

Finally, we can sometimes avoid assaults altogether by taking simple precautions.

Be Cautious

Many everyday activities may be a source of danger with some patients. Tying the shoelace of a confused elderly person, for

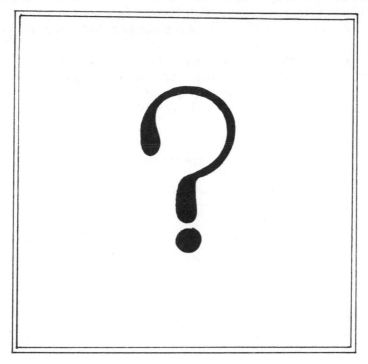

Picture 27 Do something surprising

example, puts the nurse at risk of a kick in the face without warning (picture 28). Never bend down in front of someone in such circumstances unless you are totally confident about your safety, but rather stand at the side of the patient while putting his socks and shoes on. In other circumstances you may be hit, bitten, kicked, scratched or head-butted. If you think that any particular patient is likely to be aggressive, stay alert and do not hesitate to ask for assistance or, indeed, to lend it.

Remember, to be effective, the above breakaway techniques need to be done quickly and without warning. Their purpose is to allow you to escape, and they are designed to obtain escape with the least possible harm to the attacker. It should be emphasised that each manœuvre will be most effective when it has been practised, as this will help perfect skills and build confidence in using them.

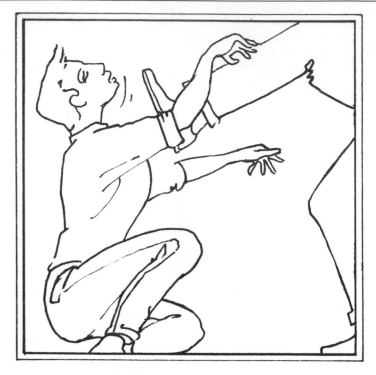

Picture 28 Be cautious

THREATS WITH WEAPONS

A wide range of weapons may be encountered, including chairs, ashtrays, knives and guns. Items of everyday ward equipment should, as far as possible, be selected to minimise their effectiveness as weapons. Light, aluminium ashtrays, plastic drinking glasses and unbreakable crockery are examples of suitable ward equipment. All are less painful than alternatives!

However, where a nurse is confronted by a threat from someone with a weapon, the following points should be borne in mind. The seriousness of the threat should first be carefully assessed. It may be possible to persuade the other person to lay down the weapon, but it will sometimes be necessary to comply without question. Your personal safety comes first: if the attacker holds a knife to your throat and demands the drug cabinet keys, hand them over quickly.

If 'talking over' seems feasible several principles are important:

- Always keep the weapon in sight.
- Ask the person (politely) to lay the weapon down. You might

say that you would find it easier to talk if the weapon were put down.

- Keep a safe distance between yourself and the other person.
- Be ready to grab an object (a chair, an umbrella or a plantpot, for example) to protect yourself should an attack occur.
- Do not turn your back on the other person.
- Note exits or other possible escape routes; surreptitiously try to get as close as possible to one.
- Be ready to shout for help or otherwise raise the alarm.

In situations where the person is known to be dangerous and violence is thought likely, police assistance should be called for.

Further Reading

Morrison C (1984) Basics in self-defence. *Community Outlook*, 80 (41): 360–1. (Briefly illustrates ways to increase confidence and reduce the risks of personal attack.)
Quinn K (1983) *Stand your Ground*. London: Orbis. (Geared especially to women's needs and partly based on one of the martial arts, this is a fairly comprehensive guide to self-defence.)

Points of Contact

The National Boards for Nursing, Midwifery and Health Visiting should be able to provide the addresses of those establishments which currently run National Board courses in the management of aggressive behaviour. However, they may not be aware of local expertise (e.g. mental health nurses) that could be utilised and even tailored to specific needs on request. The in-service training officer may already have contact with local experts and, in any case, should be made aware of the demand.

8
The Legal Position

Key Points

- It is an offence to ill-treat or wilfully neglect a patient.

- The use of force may be illegal except where the law specifically permits it.

- 'Medical treatment' normally includes nursing and may be given compulsorily to patients detained under the Mental Health Act 1983 (Part IV).

- Some protection exists for any person acting 'in good faith'.

- Force can be used without consent in certain circumstances.

- The legal position on aggression can be summed up as follows:
  Any nurse finding that a patient is behaving in a way likely to cause an imminent danger to him or herself, to others or to property, can use reasonable force to prevent this happening.

- The law should feature prominently in teaching programmes and management discussions.

At this point, it is worth reviewing the position in law of nurses who are involved in aggressive incidents. There is little information on this topic in most of the literature dealing with the problem, possibly because the law is so complex and it is easier to avoid the issue than risk misinforming the reader. We, too, are conscious of this latter possibility, but feel that a little perseverance to confront the legal jargon will allay much anxiety over what the law actually says. With this in mind, this chapter gives an overview of the relevant legalities; the reader is reminded that greater appreciation of them will follow from debate with colleagues. Note that the following discussion applies equally to the management of aggression in general health and psychiatric health care settings.

One problem with the law is that it does not always explain clearly how far staff may go in dealing with aggressive patients. It goes without saying that the nurse does not have a free hand to do whatever he or she pleases. Prior to 1983 a major shortcoming of legislation was that it was vague in many respects. Staff were often unclear about the limits of their powers and patients probably suffered abuse as a result, particularly where their freedom was concerned. One aim of the Mental Health Act 1983, then, was to go some way towards specifying what exactly might be seen as legitimate treatment and care. In this way, the Act protects nurses from overstepping the mark, but it must be remembered that the patient is also protected, and even this legislation does not always override common law. Section 127 of the Mental Health Act 1983 makes explicit the possibility that not everything a nurse might do to a patient is acceptable in law; this section states directly that it is an offence to ill-treat or wilfully neglect a patient. There is also scope for a patient or his or her representative(s) to sue for negligence if a nurse appears to have failed in his or her duties to protect the patient from harm. Even in situations where no prosecution is brought, a nurse who, by act or omission, compromises the condition or safety of a patient could be subject to the disciplinary process of the UKCC (United Kingdom Central Council for Nursing, Midwifery and Health Visiting, 1984).

What constitutes ill-treatment is important. The fundamental principles in law for nurses always to inwardly acknowledge relate to battery and assault. Under common law, any direct and intentional application of force to another person without lawful justification is battery. In the health care setting, battery might even include the use of mechanical restraint or sedation (Gostin, 1986) or forcibly searching a patient. Often, these measures can be justified, but nurses should appraise themselves of the possible limitations to actions like these. We are within the law only when there is lawful justification for the action. Assault occurs, according to common law, where someone suffers 'reasonable fear or apprehension of the use of force', and in one case an assault was said to have taken place as a patient experienced the threat of restraint when staff openly drew up a sedative injection (Townley vs Rushworth, 1964; quoted in Gostin, 1986). In addition, it is useful to bear in mind the notion of false imprisonment. This is defined as the total and unlawful restraint of a person's liberty or movement. It usually involves an assault or battery as well, although liberty may be curtailed simply by refusing to unlock a door for an informal patient. However, false imprisonment need not be maintained by the use of physical barriers, so where a patient is led to believe that a door is locked, the law may still define that a person has been imprisoned. False imprisonment also exists where the authority to detain has expired.

It has already been shown that therapeutic responses to aggression can involve some form of force, and the mechanisms whereby the nurse may be protected in law while employing these methods are introduced here. Perhaps the simplest justification for the use of force is when the patient gives consent, which may be given in writing or verbally. The use of time out procedures, as incorporated in the care plan and negotiated with the patient, would have the patient's consent. Consent can also be implied, for example, by gesture and conduct, or even by the absence of resistance to an act ordinarily expected in the course of the nurse–patient relationship (Gostin, 1986). This may, in some circumstances, provide the lawful justification for preventing an informal patient from leaving the sanctuary of the hospital. The scope enabled by these points should be tempered, however, with the knowledge that consent can be withdrawn at any time, which, in the case of the informal patient in seclusion, then produces a false imprisonment. Note also that written consent can be verbally revoked.

Nurses generally appreciate that mental health legislation enables force to be used against the will of a mentally disordered person in certain circumstances. Under the Mental Health Act 1983 (Part IV), the administration of medical treatment without consent is justified. Section 145 stipulates that 'medical treatment' includes 'nursing, as well as care, habilation and rehabilitation under medical supervision'. This extends legal cover to many other health care professionals, providing that they are acting under medical supervision. Note, though, that Part IV of the Act relates only to certain types of compulsory detention; force would not generally be permitted before an application for compulsory admission had been completed or before the holding power (section 5) had been exercised. Furthermore, the term 'treatment' is distinguished from the terms 'control' and 'management' under the Act. This prompts Gostin to point out that sedating a patient for the purpose of control and restraint should, therefore, be viewed as physical restraint rather than medical treatment. This is not to say that physical restraint is illicit. It is almost certain that any reasonable form of 'control and discipline' that is necessary for the health, safety or medical treatment of a compulsorily detained patient would be upheld by the courts (Gostin, 1986). The apparent open-endedness of the law at times is designed to prevent abuse of patients, and nurses who practise in a professional way have little to fear. Gostin concludes that where carers' professional judgements have not been possible, for example in emergency situations, the courts are likely to define 'reasonableness' in the nurse's favour. It is probably safe here, also, to borrow the *obiter dictum* from Justice Holmes: 'Detached reflection cannot be demanded in the presence of an uplifted knife' (Brown *vs* the United States; quoted in Gostin, 1986). Furthermore, where compulsorily detained patients are concerned, Section 139 of the Mental Health Act 1983 protects any person in pursuance of the Act as long as this was done in good faith and with reasonable care. This section even gives some protection when a nurse is mistaken about his or her authority to act or is mistaken about what the law says. Note, though, that Section 139 does not generally apply to informal patients.

Despite the apparent tendency of the law to favour nurses when force is applied, it is not mental health legislation that offers protection for nurses in every situation they may encounter. There are several other legal processes that can be utilised to provide the grounds for applying force (i.e. restraining) without consent. These are based in common law and in the Criminal Law Act 1967, and it is to these that we now turn.

- The *'doctrine of necessity'*. This can be used where it will immediately lead to the preservation of life. If restraint is used, it must be necessary and not just convenient, for example where restraint suits only management purposes, and the force used must be the minimum amount needed to prevent immediate danger. It is necessary to point out that, in legal parlance, restraint manifests itself in various forms. The locking of a door to prevent a confused person wandering off is seen as restraint and, as such, could constitute false imprisonment and all that entails. However, if it was immediately necessary to prevent an incompetent person from coming to any obvious and significant harm, the doctrine of necessity would probably protect the nurse in a court of law.
- *Preventing a crime*. Under the Criminal Law Act 1967, any citizen may use reasonable force either to make an arrest or to prevent a crime. Where nurses are concerned, a crime might involve a theft or an attack on a fellow patient for example, and ·

could be in progress or about to be committed. However, there is no provision here to justify retaliation or punishment once the offence has been committed, so secluding a patient as punishment afterwards would be illegal. Gostin (1986) notes that, while mental disorder may preclude the application of criminal law, any nurse acting in a reasonable fashion would probably be protected under common law.

- Preventing a breach of the peace. This is said to occur whenever harm is done or is likely to be done to a person or, in his presence, to property, or where a person is in fear of being harmed through an assault, an affray, a riot, unlawful assembly or other disturbance. Anyone seeing a breach of the peace or someone threatening the same can use reasonable force to make that person stop. In common law, this is actually everyone's duty, so fellow patients or ancillary staff could be expected to do their part as well, especially in the protection of another person. At ward level, it may be unrealistic to expect direct help from, for example, ancillary staff, but it is good practice to ensure that every member of each staff group is instructed, at least, to call for help should they see an incident of this kind. (This position is complicated where wards and departments do not enjoy regular ancillary staff who can identify themselves as members of the team.)
- Self-defence. Under this doctrine, any person can take all reasonable steps to ensure that he or she does not come to harm and that harm does not befall another: in the eyes of the law, self-defence can be carried out on behalf of someone else. Self-defence can be used to discourage or prevent unlawful force and to avoid or escape from unlawful detention, although it is important that one demonstrates to the aggressor that there is no desire to fight – a 'willingness to disengage', in the jargon. As before, the force used must not exceed that which is thought necessary in the circumstances.

The discussion above could be summed up as follows:

Any nurse finding that a patient is behaving in a way likely to cause an imminent danger to him or herself, to others or to property, can use reasonable force to prevent this happening.

The law gives the term 'reasonable' the rider that the force used is actually necessary. This suggests that if a patient can usually be dealt with by non-physical means (talking over), the use of physical restraint would constitute an assault. In addition, the force used must be proportionate to the harm to be avoided (do not use a sledgehammer to crack a nut). The degree and duration of force or restraint must also be proportionate to the harm that is being avoided.

The day-to-day application of this principle may be aided by considering the following points before engaging the aggressor with force:

- What are the aims of using force in this situation?
- Are these aims justified in law?
- Is it reasonable for force to be used in the first place?
- What is the least amount of force needed to contain the situation?
- What measures will need to be taken to continue safe management when restraint is discontinued?

Some of these points could be discussed during the formulation of the care plan. They should certainly reflect the departmental philosophy and be professionally acceptable to nursing colleagues. The wisdom of the medical and other multidisciplinary team members should also be sought, because action faithful to a common aim of care should be unanimously supported.

Finally, although relatively little space has been allocated to the legal aspect of care, the reader should not take this as a reflection of its importance to good working practice. Nurses, as individuals, should make themselves fully aware of the legal considerations of their responses to aggression, and a concise further reading list is included below to help with this. Law is also made daily, through legal judgments and precedents, so it is interesting to read the journals and newspapers to keep fully up to date. Furthermore, nursing management should be lobbied locally to provide detailed advice and guidance for staff on professional, ethical and legal issues. Where necessary, management should also be asked to create appropriate training opportunities. Addressing these matters is an essential next step in equipping oneself for demonstrating accountability.

Further Reading

Department of Health (1990) *Code of Practice: Mental Health Act 1983.* London: HMSO. (An essential accompaniment to good practice, this book clarifies most of the issues not properly addressed by the Act itself. Produced after pressure from groups, including MIND.)

Gostin L (1983) *A Practical Guide to Mental Health Law.* London: MIND. (A very digestible version of the legislation.)

Hoggett B (1990) *Mental Health Law*, 3rd edn. London: Sweet & Maxwell. (Positively *the* definitive tome on this branch of the law and a very comprehensive source of law relating to aggression.)

9
Action to Take Following Incidents of Aggression

Key Points

- Aggression may be more common than statistics suggest, because many staff choose not to document incidents.

- Supportive management may be needed before aggression is reported properly.

- All incidents of aggression should be reported so that an objective assessment of staff risk can be made, and recording is vital where staff (or patients) may wish to make a formal complaint.

- A detailed report should be made on any incident.

- Guidelines should be given to staff, outlining the kinds of incident they should report.

- Staff involved in aggressive encounters need understanding and support; even 'petty' incidents can have long-term consequences.

- The need for support groups and, sometimes, specialist counselling should be acknowledged.

- The needs of the aggressor and bystanders should also be considered; their views may provide valuable insights into the reasons for the incident.

RECORDING INCIDENTS OF AGGRESSION

Although it is unclear whether or not aggression towards staff is in fact increasing, the problem of aggression is now well recognised. A recent Health and Safety Commission survey suggested that nurses working in psychiatric and Accident and Emergency Departments were most likely to be the recipients of aggression. The survey showed that 1 in 200 workers (nurses and other health service employees) had suffered a major injury following a violent attack during the preceding year. One in every 21 workers had been threatened with a weapon, and more than 1 in 6 had been verbally threatened (Health Services Advisory Committee, 1987). These findings may be an underestimate of the extent of aggression experienced by staff, as there is evidence that staff may be under-reporting incidents (Haller and Deluty, 1988).

ACTIVITY 9

List the reasons why incidents of aggression may be under-reported.
Now see the discussion below.

Discussion
Incidents of aggression may be under-reported for several reasons. Drummond et al (1989) suggest that staff may be unwilling to report incidents because they believe such reporting would amount to an admission of professional failure, particularly if they work in an area where violence is uncommon. It may be that staff fear being labelled by colleagues as incompetent and/or that they do not want their skills to be called into question at the expense of other considerations. Some staff may fail to report incidents because they think colleagues will be unsympathetic: Lanza (1984) reports nurses as feeling unsupported by colleagues following incidents of assault. Although these nurses wanted to attend to their own needs rather than to those of the patient who assaulted them, many nurses felt it unprofessional to express their feelings.

Another possible reason for non-reporting is that staff may fail to acknowledge the seriousness of the incident. Lanza (1983) suggests that nursing staff may, following incidents of aggression, suppress their reactions as a means of protecting themselves from overwhelming anxiety and helplessness. Di Bella (1979) cites the case of one staff member who said, just before being severely beaten by a patient, 'He is just misunderstood. He would never hurt me'. It may also be that some staff do not report incidents as they see them as part of the job; as one colleague put it, 'Well, you expect to get hit working in this place'.

Under-reporting may also occur because staff have not agreed on what they consider to be tolerable aggression. Without some idea of what is acceptable, inconsistency will arise over what to report. There is a suggestion that 'petty' acts of aggression may number up to four times those reported. Our own anecdotal evidence indicates that verbal abuse and harassment are indeed under-reported, as is racial and sexual harassment. Interestingly, the Trades Union Congress (1988) asserts that the latter two forms of harassment are also forms of aggression.

ACTIVITY 10

At this point you might like to compare your views on tolerable aggression in the work setting with those of colleagues.

Finally, under-reporting may be due to the fact that student nurses are one of the most likely target groups to be aggressed against (possibly as a result of their high number of patient contact hours compared to trained staff and their relative lack of experience in responding to patient aggression). Student nurses may fear loss of face if they trouble staff with their concerns, and they may be given the impression by some senior staff that they should 'put it down to experience'. With the increased supervision of student nurses envisaged in Project 2000 courses, it will be interesting to see how things change in this area.

No staff member should feel afraid to report incidents, and nurse managers have a crucial role to play here in encouraging open discussion on these issues. Without clear guidelines and supportive nursing management, staff members will tend to be overly concerned about management reacting unfavourably to reports of aggression (Drummond et al 1989).

Without a formal record of reporting incidents of aggression (both physical and verbal), it is not possible to be objective about the number of acts of aggression or about which locations are the most dangerous, and monitoring the effectiveness of preventive programmes would be impossible. This is important because managers have a statutory duty to identity the nature and extent of risks their employees face. In cases where employees might wish to claim for compensation and where prosecution is considered, it is essential that incidents are recorded. The recording system should ensure that:

- a written record is made soon after the event;
- information is gathered from all concerned;
- details of victim(s) and aggressor(s) are recorded, including name, age, sex, address and telephone number, whether patient or staff and whether on or off duty;
- an account is given of what happened before, during and after

the incident, including actions taken to prevent a recurrence, details of any injury, details of location (including the name of the ward or department as appropriate) of the incident. Line drawings, if necessary for clarity, and the time of the incident are recorded.

- the report document is signed by its author;
- a procedure for informing the personnel and occupational health departments is followed;
- the incidents can later be subjected to statistical analysis of, for example, incident, seriousness, location and personnel involved. To facilitate such analysis a suitable retrieval system should be used;
- guidelines are provided so that staff are aware of what incidents should be recorded. It is impossible to be specific about what to record as people vary in what they regard as worthy of recording. As mentioned above, many staff feel reluctance to report incidents as they see them as part of the job or feel that colleagues will be unsympathetic (Lanza, 1984). It is important that opportunity and encouragement is given to air such views; this will also help to achieve some measure of consistency in reporting. The following guidelines are suggested:

  (i) Any incident involving injury by another to him or herself and/or to others should be reported, as should

 (ii) incidents involving physical restraint,

(iii) incidents resulting in seclusion of the patient, and

(iv) incidents that involve damage to property.

 (v) Allegations of any of the above incidents should be recorded prior to investigation.

(vi) Incidents involving threats and verbal abuse can be recorded in the patient's notes and also in the ward/department incident report book. There should be a procedure for informing others involved in the patient's care, which may include the patient's relatives, particularly if the patient is likely to visit or live with them. Of course, this breach of professional confidence should only be considered if it is thought to be in the patient's best interest and/or is seen to protect others. As far as possible, the patient's cooperation should be sought prior to the disclosure of information to a third party; only in exceptional circumstances should the patient's wishes be ignored (Health Services Advisory Committee, 1987).

COUNSELLING HELP AND SUPPORT FOR STAFF

For most people, being involved in an aggressive incident is stressful, and people cope with such stress in a variety of ways. Some people manage to retain an air of outward composure, while others enter a state of shock. For some, difficulties arise some time after the event. The range of emotions felt is also varied: some feel a great loss of self-esteem and may blame themselves for the incident, whereas others may feel hostile towards the aggressor and seek retribution. Furthermore, it is not just following 'serious' incidents that staff require most help. Some staff react very badly, and so-called petty assaults can cause symptoms consistent with a diagnosis of post-traumatic stress disorder for weeks after the incident (Whittington and Wykes, 1989, 1992). The point here is that people involved in aggressive encounters need understanding and support, and, for some, long-term counselling may be required both before and on returning to work. Nurses, perhaps, may need extra encouragement to seek help following incidents, as they are more used to seeing themselves as givers of care rather than receivers of help. Therefore, it is important that the work situation is receptive to staff concerns. Managers, in particular, can be effective in fostering a supportive and caring environment for staff by implementing policies that offer staff the opportunity to discuss their needs. In Whittington and Wykes (1989), staff expressed a need to talk about the incident and wanted their hurt and anger acknowledged, some wanting to go over the incident to see if they did the right thing, others preferring a formal group to discuss their feelings. A frequent request was relief from being with patients: time off the ward for as little as 10 minutes was a popular option. Whittington and Wykes suggest in a recent study (1992) that it may be beneficial to educate nurses about how they might feel if they were involved in a violent incident. The notion that this would improve the ability to deal with the psychological effects of violence is in keeping with the concept of emotional inoculation (Janis, 1958), which is said to be effective because the 'work of worrying' is done in advance. Counselling help may also be delivered through locally organised support sessions by colleagues. Where these are not enough and extended support is required, staff should have access to a counsellor with specialist knowledge of the care context. In cases where a staff member may want to bring a private prosecution or seek compensation, help or advice may be sought from the line manager, personnel department, staff organisations and outside legal advisors.

COUNSELLING HELP AND SUPPORT FOR THE AGGRESSOR

From the aggressor's point of view, the incident may have been entirely appropriate or, alternatively, he or she may feel acute shame and embarrassment. As far as possible the aggressor's views should be sought, as they may provide valuable insights into the incident. In some cases, the seriousness of the incident may require the police to be called in to remove the aggressor, and it may not be possible or appropriate to discuss the incident with him or her. Fortunately, the majority of incidents are not this serious, and an understanding approach is required in order to help the aggressor face up to his or her behaviour. The type of help and support he or she may need can include a frank discussion with staff concerning their expectations and the consequences should further aggression arise, and involvement in a long-term programme to control aggression.

COUNSELLING HELP AND SUPPORT FOR THOSE NOT DIRECTLY INVOLVED

Witnesses to aggression may react in a number of ways. A junior colleague, perhaps experiencing patient aggression for the first time, may be shocked and fearful for his or her future safety. Patients and bystanders may misunderstand what is happening and become upset. As far as possible, bystanders should be kept informed of what is happening and told how they can help. Following incidents of aggression, nurses should talk to witnesses to ascertain their views, explain the recent event and find out what further help may be required.

It is important that an incident of aggression is seen as an issue for the aggressee, the aggressor and even the bystanders.

Further Reading

Murray M G and Snyder J C (1991) When staff are assaulted. *Journal of Psychosocial Nursing*, **29** (7): 24–9. (Describes how a nursing consultation support service was set up, and makes a number of suggestions for evaluating such a service.)

Richards D (1989) Hidden scars. *Nursing Times*, **85** (22): 65–8. (Describes the help offered to women following violent attacks.)

Rose J and Richards D (1991) Healing the mind. *Nursing Times*, **87** (14): 40–2.

Useful Addresses

National Association for Staff Support
9 Caradon Close
Woking
Surrey GU21 3DU
(Can provide information on counselling services in your area and also has guidelines on setting up support services for staff.)

Compensation schemes:

NHS Injury Benefits Scheme
Superannuation Division
Department of Health
Hesketh House
200 Broadway
Fleetwood
Lancashire RY7 8LG

The Criminal Injuries Compensation Board
10/12 Russell Square
London WC1B 5EN

Comments:

Few nurses pursue claims with the CICB, perhaps because of the lengthy delays in achieving any outcome. The facility exists and should be used if only to establish the extent of the need.

Part III
REVIEW

This part of the book is concerned with the final stage of the cycle of nursing experience of aggression. Having given thought to assessing, planning and carrying out the various nursing approaches to aggressive behaviour, we here evaluate those approaches. The key word is REVIEW.

A major aim of any review is to provide opportunities for learning. By sharing thoughts and feelings, by considering our own experiences and those of others, by highlighting shortcomings and by praising individual strengths, the quality of our nursing care can be improved when meeting similar situations in the future. Also included here

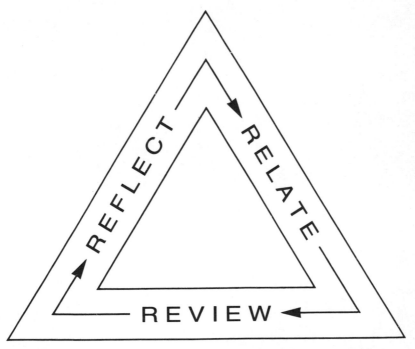

Figure 10.1 A model for the management of aggressive behaviour

is a consideration of personal risk and how steps can be taken to avoid this. An element of the review process we envisage compares with Schon's (1983) ideas about reflective observation, which he sees as resulting in the development of personal theory, which could be thought of as theory derived from experience.

The process of review merges with stage one of the next cycle, since a period of reflective observation follows one experience and precedes the next. The subjects of both chapters in Part III can be seen as completing the cycle and linking one cycle to the next.

10
Incident Analysis

Key Points

- Careful review of each incident provides a valuable learning opportunity; those things done well and those not done well can be put in perspective.

- An 'ABCD' analysis provides a useful framework for reviewing incidents.

- Clinical supervision can be used to review therapeutic performance in the management of aggression.

- Standard setting and quality circles can be used to monitor the effectiveness and quality of nursing care.

The idea of evaluation is an integral part of the learning process. In relation to the nursing of individuals who have displayed aggressive behaviour, it is possible to carry out several types of evaluation of the care given. Firstly, it is sometimes helpful to spend some time alone carrying out a personal review of events. In particularly busy settings or periods, this may be all that can be achieved. Although personal reflections should not be accepted as a complete substitute for any other form of review, they are a vital starting point for the reflective practitioner. Secondly, and by far the most important review process, is that which takes place within a group. This context enables a number of people, not only those who are taking part, to benefit from the lessons to be learned. It also allows junior staff to benefit from the clinical expertise and experience of more senior staff, whether or not they were involved. Thirdly, there may occasionally, be reason for incident review to take a more formal line. For example, where aggressive behaviour could have serious implications, management may wish to hold some sort of enquiry. High standards of nursing practice in relation to aggression, and careful record keeping at all times, should pose few problems for this type of review.

Our main concern in discussing incident analysis is in encouraging the greater use of analysis, especially in groups, so that nursing approaches to aggression may be improved. We advocate what might be called an ABCD analysis, in which each letter provides a convenient prompt for the stages of reviewing Antecedents, Behaviours, Consequences and Decisions. In each of the sections below certain questions are suggested to help structure the discussion that takes place. Some of these questions may in the first instance, be more suited to personal review than discussion.

A – ANTECEDENTS

This stage requires the group (or individual) to think about the situation that seemed to precede the aggressive episode. The rationale is that the material highlighted may heighten awareness of the cause of the episode, and the knowledge gained will guide responses to avoid similar problems in any future recurrence.

Questions for consideration include:

- What seemed to lead up to the incident?
- What appeared to be the aggressor's motives?
- What was going on at the time?
- What did particular individuals say and do?
- What were others doing?
- How did I feel?
- How was the aggressor feeling, and how do I know this?
- What structural factors may have had a bearing on the incident, e.g. is the routine too strict?
- Were any warnings given?
- With hindsight, how predictable was this episode?

B – BEHAVIOURS

Reviewing behaviours involves a careful reconstruction of the actual event. As many perspectives as possible should be gathered. Care should be taken to *describe* the behaviours of those involved and not to make inferences from these behaviours at this stage.

Questions for consideration include:

- What exactly did the aggressor do?
- What was the aggressor's body language?

- Was he or she hitting out or making threatening remarks?
- What did I or other staff say and do (including body language)?
- Did the aggressor say anything during the incident (comments made may provide a clue to the reason for the behaviour)?
- Were any other patients or other people implicated in any way?
- Was any aspect of the incident minimised by the preventative actions?

C – CONSEQUENCES

This stage requires a description of the outcomes of the episode, as well as an indication of the suitability or desirability of the outcomes.

Questions for consideration include:

- How did we react?
- Whose safety was compromised?
- How did the episode finally come to an end?
- Was this a satisfactory outcome in the circumstances?
- What did we want to achieve and what was the actual outcome?
- Were our actions therapeutic and professional?
- Did staff feel secure and happy in the actions taken to gain control of the situation?
- How do I feel now?
- Is the incident likely to happen again?
- With hindsight, should we have behaved differently?

D – DECISIONS

This could be seen as a review of the review, but also involves the formulation of initiatives on the part of the team or the leadership for taking further, for example, with management. Whatever the outcome of the review, there will usually be something that could form the basis of an action plan to facilitate development of the nursing policy on the management of aggression within the particular clinical unit.

Questions for consideration include:

- Do we have an acceptable and suitable mechanism for analysis to take place?
- How easy was it to involve the right people in the analysis?
- What decisions need to be made now that the incident has been discussed?
- Do we need to change any aspects of the present policy for dealing with aggression?

- Do we have adequate nursing and medical support and how will this subject be broached?
- Do we need to change the patient's plan of care?
- Were there any ward design or ward routine aspects of the incident that should be addressed?
- What ongoing help do the victim and aggressor need, and do these facilities exist or need setting up or improving?
- What issues need to be addressed by management?
- What have I learned that I will bring to future encounters?

A private area of the ward is important for the review to take place, and there should be an atmosphere of support and understanding. It is vital that it should be seen as a learning opportunity, and in no way should it emulate an inquisition. Staff should not be made to feel they have failed. Wherever possible, the review should take place soon after an incident. While those involved in the review are away, the ward might be covered by those staff who were not on duty when the incident took place, or, alternatively, it may be necessary to arrange staff cover from another ward to enable the group process to occur without interruption. Inevitably, holding the review will prove more difficult than letting an important opportunity pass; remember that if you do not make the effort to make it happen, you will never know what could have been learned.

At the beginning, an unstructured approach may be appropriate, especially if it is thought necessary to convince those taking part that the intention is to be constructive. One way to start might be to ask staff for their initial reactions. This often highlights the areas needing the most urgent attention. For example, a staff member may want to talk about his or her feelings of resentment towards the aggressor. Such immediate responses are relevant to the more structured discussion to follow. Care should also be taken to see that staff feel able to explore the areas in which the incident was not so well managed. Of course, there should be adequate review of the positive aspects of the episode as well, to give credit where credit is due. Views from the aggressor, if appropriate, and from any relevant witnesses will provide further insights. Finally, it is important that *all* incidents are carefully reviewed. The petty incident that was well managed can serve as a valuable learning opportunity, especially as this can be discussed in less fraught surroundings. Here, the main focus could be on the interpersonal skills used by the nurse.

The emphasis above is on the group orientation of review, but there is an increasing expectation nowadays that nurses will reflect on and review their experiences by themselves. The group review is important, for example, because it may lead to changes in unit policy, which affects everybody, but nursing is carried out by individuals at the personal level, and in the final analysis the changes have to be made at the personal level. This means that some sort of personal review is called for – reflective practice. The questions above provide the basis of the form that such reflection could take, but we would encourage individuals to ask other questions and elaborate on the ones above according to the needs of the circumstances. Personal reflection requires an understanding of the process and a chance, periodically, to share one's reflections with others. The group process outlined above and the processes described below can complement this activity.

Incident analysis and review can fulfil several purposes apart from those focused on above, which involve checking how well systems work and capitalising on the learning opportunities afforded by the management of aggressive behaviour. Staff support has been discussed in an earlier chapter, and will always be necessary. The need for support may only become clear when staff come together in a group. This may be because an individual has hidden her or his reactions to the episode, and nobody has previously noticed any untoward effect, or it may be that the analysis brings back the shocking memories of what happened. Those participating in the group should be sensitive to this prospect. The staff affected may not always be those who were directly involved, as it seems that, for some, the fear of being involved in aggression is just as unsettling as the actuality. However, apart from the immediate staff issues, review provides an important opportunity for monitoring standards of care given; some examples of the form this could take are included below.

Personal standards will be considered first. The value of reflection has been noted above, but review of an aggressive encounter could be encompassed in other activities. One review mechanism already widely used in mental health nursing is clinical supervision. Here, a practitioner reviews her or his ongoing clinical work and relevant aspects of his or her own reactions to that work. This is carried out in collaboration with a colleague who is at least equally skilled (Minot and Adamski, 1989). The aims of supervision are the patient's clinical improvement and the practitioner's professional development. Minot and Adamski see self-growth in awareness and knowledge as being achieved through supervision. They also highlight the scope that clinical supervision affords the practitioner to vent frustrations and argue that it bolsters the sense of security, thus offering an important support system. In this way supervision may lessen the need for more formal counselling help in the event of the practitioner becoming the victim of aggression. The Post-Registration Education and Practice (PREP) Project's recommendation that all newly qualified nurses should have a preceptor could be seen as an opportunity to move towards the adoption of clinical supervision in settings other than mental health nursing (UKCC, 1990). After all, not only is clinical supervision a vehicle for review of our nursing practice, but it has also been asserted that it should be used fully to develop the professional self (Platt-Koch, 1986).

It is preferable for those undergoing clinical supervision to be allowed to choose their supervisor, and that the latter should agree to the request; it should be a voluntary relationship. Invariably, the supervisor will be a colleague, so it could be argued that supervision is a form of peer review. However, peer review can take a number of forms. Typically, it may consist of a group of peers (for example staff nurses) who meet to analyse a given nursing practice and make recommendations (perhaps for their own performance). There should be a facilitator, skilled in group work, who may or may not be a member of the ward team. Review by peers should enable a more open and honest exploration of the issues arising and, by implication, should be more able to foster a growth relationship because the evaluation of performance does not (directly) involve a line manager. However, the unit manager should be involved insofar as the group's conclusions and recommendations could form the basis of changes to clinical practice (Oreschnik, 1984).

One means of review and monitoring standards that could be more widely considered in mental health nursing is that of 'standard setting'. The term 'standard' denotes a measure to which others should conform or by which they should be judged, and it could be argued that the therapeutic management of aggression is highly conducive to standard setting. The idea of standard setting has been widely documented in recent years (e.g. Kitson, 1990), and basically refers to the process whereby a representative group of health care workers meet to decide what constitutes acceptable standards in relation to a specific aspect of nursing care common to the practice of those present. They do this by setting criteria, against which actual practice may be judged. The 'standard' that results indicates the 'resources' that exist to begin with (structure criteria), the actions to be carried out (process criteria) and what will be achieved (outcome criteria).

Needless to say, standards are pointless if the actual care delivered is not measured against them. It is vital, therefore, that nursing outcomes are monitored and that the staff group receives feedback. In *A Strategy for Nursing* (Department of Health, 1989), the use of standards is endorsed for all fields of nursing.

A set of standards for the management of various aggressive behaviours would, it is suggested, aim to achieve a solution to any aggressive encounter such that neither staff nor patient could suffer physical injury or harm (or such that this would be minimised), while maintaining an environment in which therapeutic nurse–patient relationships can continue. In their conception, standards must be realistic, achievable and clinically sound.

One possible criticism of incident analysis taken on its own is that it can be seen as only a reactive exercise, whereas quality circles seem to be more proactive. When these are used in industry, a group of volunteers focus on a work-related problem in an organised way. They meet weekly to develop their preferred solution to the problem and then take responsibility for selling it to the leadership. If it is accepted, they help implement it and monitor the results (Christie and O'Reilly, 1984). This kind of approach needs cautious application to the problem of nursing aggressive patients and might be better suited to some specific aspects of the problem of aggression in a given setting. However, as a management tool, it has several virtues. Firstly, it provides a way of involving all the team in planning and decision making. Secondly, it is a good example of a 'bottom-up' approach to change. It may also facilitate the personal development of those taking part, as supervisory skills are said to improve through participation in quality circles, and participants may adopt more positive attitudes. Furthermore, there may be more universal benefits. It has been suggested that the adoption of quality circles in one hospital has led to improvements in communication, a higher quality of service and increased job satisfaction (Robson, 1984).

There are a number of other activities that could be adapted and utilised in the process of analysing and evaluating nursing management of aggressive behaviours. Where the primary goal of review is the education and training of staff, an approach involving critical incident analysis has been shown to be effective, particularly with student nurses (Smith and Russell, 1991). One advantage of the method described by Smith and Russell is that the activity can be carried out some time after the event because great use is made of students' diaries and reflections. Where the experience of an incident involving aggression is more immediate, it may be more appropriate to deal with it sooner. Debriefing would be expedient in this case (Pearson and Smith, 1985), as this is recommended as a way of appreciating the learning that has taken place. It can also, of course, deliver the support that will be necessary for some students or at least show up those who need it most.

The importance of incident analysis and review can be seen from the discussion above. It may be that the method chosen is not so important, but the fact that some form of review takes place certainly is. The principle of review must be taken seriously. There are various ways of utilising experiences to improve future performance, particularly where some form of reflection is carried out. However, review also provides an opportunity for standards to be evaluated. Where this takes place, the mechanism exists for providing assurances to nursing management and the public that clinical performance in a given unit is satisfactory. Quality assurance in the therapeutic nursing management of aggressive behaviour is upon us. It may be that attention to the role of review, and responding to the changes elucidated, will be critical in enabling high standards to be achieved.

Further Reading

Health and Safety Executive (1986) *Violence to Staff: A Basis for Assessment and Prevention*. London: HMSO. (Helpful advice on monitoring the incidence of violence, which includes suggested contents for an incident form.)
Robson M (1982) *Quality Circles: A Practical Guide*. London: Gower.
Robson M (1984) *Quality Circles in Action*. London: Gower.

11
Assessing and Avoiding Personal Risk

> **Key Points**
> - All staff should consider the issue of personal safety for themselves.
> - All staff have a responsibility for their own safety.
> - Risk can be reduced, both in hospital and outside.
> - Managers have a special responsibility to provide safe working environments for their staff.

AM I AT RISK UNNECESSARILY?

In this section the reader is invited to think about how individuals can make their own working environment as safe as possible. It is an unfortunate reality that hospitals, by virtue of their large size and easy access, are conducive to high levels of theft and acts of vandalism, as well as providing the settings in which staff may be the recipients of direct violence at work. Staff residences and hospital grounds are also unsafe.

The following questions will help you think about the risks you may be facing at work.

The Risk at Work Checklist

For each question you are asked to place an X at the point on the line that best reflects your current views.

	Frequently	**Rarely**
1. I walk through the grounds alone at night	|———————————|
2. I walk down quiet corridors alone	|———————————|
3. Because of my shifts, I have to wait at bus stops alone	|———————————|

	Very	Not at all
4. The staff changing room is isolated	|———————————|	
5. My hospital accommodation is secure	|———————————|	

	Always	Never
6. In an emergency, I can get help quickly	|———————————|	
7. The ward is safely staffed	|———————————|	
8. When confronted with aggressive incidents at work, I am skilled in managing them	|———————————|	
9. I feel safe at work	|———————————|	

AVOIDING UNNECESSARY RISK

The Institutional Setting

If any of the above questions caused you to think again about your personal safety, the following suggestions will help:

- Avoid walking through the hospital grounds alone at night (and during the day if there is known risk).
- Avoid walking through quiet, isolated corridors alone, day or night.
- Promptly report poor lighting in corridors and hospital grounds, including car parks.
- Report inefficient locks on doors and windows.
- Consider carrying a personal alarm. Of course, these should be seen as adjuncts to personal safety rather than as a substitute for extra staff. Personal alarms may attract someone to assist when people are about (although this is certainly not guaranteed), but they will be of little use when isolated. If you really do feel unsafe in certain situations without a personal alarm, you should, perhaps, be asking for more staff.
- At work, whether it be a ward or an out-patient clinic, always check the identity and purpose of strangers. This can simply be done by asking if you can help them. The vast majority of

people will turn out to be there for legitimate reasons and will be happy to explain their presence. Be suspicious of someone who cannot readily account for his or her presence, and seek further advice from a colleague on your next move. Wearing a white coat is not a guarantee of legitimate presence.

- Review your emergency procedure. Ask whether it is adequate to meet present needs.
- Report inadequate staffing levels and, perhaps just as importantly, insufficient staff mix. You may, on paper, be well staffed but, in reality, the numbers may be made up of inexperienced junior colleagues who may not yet have acquired skills in aggression management or, indeed, the many other skills required for all-round effective care.
- If you have not been trained in aggression management techniques, or it has been some time since you last updated your skills, request to attend an appropriate aggression management course. If no such provision exists, remind management of your needs.

The Community Setting

Nurses who work in the community should also consider the following points.

Dangers in Patients' Homes

- Check that you have enough information about your client. Note especially whether or not your client has a history of aggression or is suffering from a condition likely to produce aggression, or whether there are difficult social circumstances.
- Leave a detailed schedule of your intended visits and their durations at work or, if after hours, with your partner or a friend. Remember that if you take your diary with you, nobody can work out where you were last. Having two diaries is a necessity.
- Call back to base after your rounds or phone to say where you are.
- Let colleagues know if you have cause for concern, and ask them to check up on your safe return by a certain time.
- Arrange a distress coding so that when you phone in, you can alert help without compromising your safety. Perhaps reference to a fictitious colleague would be a suitable choice or coding, e.g. 'It's important that I stay here longer than expected, so could you let Sister Quinn know I can't make the appointment.'

This raises the need for careful induction when temporary staff, for example receptionists, are used.

- As far as possible, work in pairs at night or when you cannot avoid visiting a client who is known to be dangerous.
- Be alert to clues in the environment that something is wrong. The patient may be abusive when he opens the door or there may be dangerous implements lying about the room. Use your judgement about when not to go in or about what is an opportune moment to leave. If in doubt, make an excuse and leave.
- Do not enter the house if the person you need to see is not there.
- In situations where you feel there is danger, try to judge whether or not the aggressor would be put off by letting him or her know that other people are going to be checking up on what has happened to you.
- Try to arrange as many meetings as possible with clients at your 'home' base, i.e. the surgery or clinic.
- Report any incident that gives you cause for concern – to the police if appropriate. Warn colleagues or other professionals who might need to call on the patient.

Dangers While Travelling to Patients' Homes

- Park where you know you can get into your car safely on your return – perhaps in a well-used, well-lit car park.
- Avoid 'advertising' your car as belonging to a community nurse: it may be broken into in search of drugs. Avoid advertising yourself, too, as you may be seen as carrying drugs. (The authors have a colleague who carries his stationery in a supermarket plastic bag and 'dresses down' when visiting some clients.)
- Consider carrying a personal alarm, a personal paging system or even a good whistle.
- Always know exactly how to get to your destination. Avoid getting lost.
- Avoid dimly lit alleyways.
- Wear shoes that are suitable for walking or running and that do not make noise.
- Lock yourself in your car as soon as you get in.
- Keep your car in good running order. Carry a can of petrol and change for the telephone.

The above are things you can do to minimise risk to yourself. However, as a manager, there are several other considerations for both the community and the institutional setting:

- Consider the use of security technology, for example intercoms for staff residences, video monitoring at key sites and wall alarms in isolated areas and high-risk working environments, such as Accident and Emergency Departments and psychiatric wards, as well as the need for personal alarms for staff and/or a paging system whereby staff can summon help in an emergency. However, security equipment should not be seen as an alternative to providing staff with therapeutic aggression management skills or as a substitute for adequate staffing levels.
- Ensure that lighting is adequate and regularly maintained throughout the hospital and grounds. Well-lit car parks and entrances to staff residences may help to deter potential attackers.
- Ensure that access to buildings is reduced to a minimum number of sites. Of course, there may be conflict here between the wish for convenience of access and the security of the building. However, it may be acceptable at night to limit access to the main entrance only.
- Ensure that door and window locks are effective.
- Ensure that there are adequate security personnel.
- Ensure that staff facilities, such as changing rooms, are secure. This may mean relocating them to a less isolated part of the hospital.
- Consider bussing staff to and from work as an alternative to staff taking public transport or walking home alone. Where staff are experiencing difficulty with local buses, it may be possible to get the bus timetable altered to be more convenient. Altering duty rotas may be another consideration; having staff rotas that begin and start at the same time throughout the hospital may help to reduce the likelihood of staff being on their own going to and coming from work.
- Encourage all staff to introduce themselves when visiting other departments.
- Ensure that wards are adequately staffed with the right skill mix and that there is an ongoing training programme in aggression management skills.
- Where staff conduct late evening clinics, consider the implications of this: a lone individual is more vulnerable to attack.
- Provide all staff with, at the very least, an information pack on the management of aggression. Martin (1984) reported that staff found that training and managerial support were more useful than just giving them guidelines.
- When planning services, ensure that any resource implications,

either in terms of equipment or more staff, for providing safe working conditions are budgeted for right from the beginning.

- Have a yearly survey, perhaps in the form of a questionnaire, to ascertain staff views on security issues.
- Ensure that the possibility of aggression is taken seriously by staff and not dismissed on the basis that 'it never happens to you'.
- Support the decisions of staff. They should not be made to feel guilty for cutting short a meeting or visit where they sense danger.

Many readers will, no doubt, say that the above recommendations are all right in theory but that the reality of the practice situation makes them more akin to aims. Inadequate staffing levels and lack of funds frequently create the main obstacles. This state of affairs cannot be denied, but employees have the right to a safe working environment. It is imperative, therefore, that all members of staff take the responsibility for those things that they can do to protect themselves and assiduously voice their concern about those aspects of the working environment that are beyond individual control. Managers, likewise, have a responsibility to *provide* safe working environments for their staff. The onus is on nursing managers to gain an awareness of staff needs as perceived by staff themselves and then provide the necessary resources to meet those needs.

ASSESSING THE PROBABILITY OF AGGRESSION

It seemed fitting to conclude this book with a short discussion on the prediction of aggression. Prediction is part and parcel of everyday life, and accurate prediction of aggression would have enormous benefits for us as professionals. If it were possible to say who will become aggressive and in what situations aggression will occur, steps could presumably be taken to limit the course. With our present state of knowledge, however, it is not generally possible to predict, with a high degree of accuracy, individual instances of aggression. It has been shown that there are a tremendous number of factors to be considered in each encounter, so it might be better to talk in terms of the probability of aggression occurring when certain conditions prevail. Weather forecasting provides a good analogy because, here, guarantees are rarely given. Forecasters are often more or less accurate for the country as a whole, but they cannot be certain of the weather at a given time in a particular place. Like nurses, weather forecasters lack an adequate model to enable accurate predictions. In social science, it is easier to predict the behaviour of groups than that of an individual. It is possible to estimate reasonably accurately the total number of violent deaths that will take place next year, but nobody can say who will be the victims of such crimes. Of course, the more information available about an individual, the more certainly his or her future behaviour can be predicted. It is likely that greater accuracy could be achieved in estimating the possibility of a violent death for armed robbers than for vicars, for example. The checklist below is designed to provide a framework for estimating the probability that aggression will occur during an interaction. It includes a selection of items that are probably relevant for many sorts of health care setting, although the list is not exhaustive and the reader may wish to add other points pertinent to his or her particular circumstances.

The more often you agree with or answer YES to the following statements, the greater the likelihood of aggression.

Characteristics of the Nurse

- I have not had experience in handling aggressive incidents in the past.
- I have not had training in aggression management skills.
- I do not have the interpersonal skills to defuse aggressive encounters.
- I tend to lose control of my thoughts and feelings in aggressive situations.
- I do not know the person very well.
- I am the bearer of unwelcome news for the person.
- I have to perform an intervention that he or she will find unpleasant and/or resent.
- I feel very uncomfortable in this situation.
- This person scares me.

Characteristics of the Other Person

- He or she shows verbal and non-verbal signs of being angry.
- He or she has been aggressive in the past.
- He or she has been aggressive towards me in the past.
- He or she is angry at being ill.
- He or she is showing signs of severe distress.
- He or she is intoxicated.
- He or she is on drugs.
- He or she is confused.

- He or she is in pain.
- He or she has a mental illness.
- He or she is getting more worked up the longer I stay.
- He or she perceives me as a threat of some sort.

Characteristics of the Environment

- There are weapons or other clues in the environment that I find threatening.
- Others are inciting him or her to aggress.
- There is an audience that the person wants to impress.
- The environment is noisy.
- Staff have poor communication skills.
- There are few facilities.

Note that the risk of serious injury is greater when:

- working alone;
- help is not readily available;
- your escape route is blocked;
- you lack the skills to fend off an attack.

If you perceive the probability of aggression to be high, there are at least three options to consider. Firstly, discuss your concerns with your line manager. This will enable clarification of your needs and raise the issue of how best they can be met. Secondly, use the information to prepare yourself for the possibility of trouble. To be forewarned is to be forearmed. It is not always practical to avoid interacting with patients who are known to be a high risk, but, in these situations, we can make preparations beforehand so that, for instance, help can be summoned quickly should the situation get out of hand. Thirdly, it may be appropriate to inform colleagues of your concerns, particularly if you agreed with any of the items under 'characteristics of the other' in the above list.

There is, however, a caveat: a potentially violent occasion can arise when only one or two of the above pointers are present. For instance, the clue that impending aggression might be near is sometimes signalled only by a raised voice.

Further Reading

Blair D T and New S A (1991) Assaultive behaviour: know the risks. *Journal of Psychosocial Nursing*, **29** (11): 25–30. (A useful analysis of risk factors, which highlights the part played by knowing and unknowing staff provocation.)

Health and Safety Commission (1974) Health and Safety at Work etc. Act, 1974; *The Act Outlined* (HSC 3), *Advice to Employers* (HSC 4) and *Advice to Employees* (HSC 5). London: HMSO. (Detailed guidance for everyone on the implications of the Act for working practices.)

Lamplugh D (1988) *Beating Aggression: A Practical Guide for Working Women*. London: Weidenfeld and Nicolson. (A very detailed guide to personal safety, with many good tips for eluding the dangers one may find in the community.)

Appendix
Prevention: an Overview

P Prepare yourself. Ask yourself how long it has been since you reviewed your skills. When did you last attend a workshop or course? If a manager asks, how informed are you of your staff's needs?

R Review workplace policy. Ask whether it is adequate to meet present needs. Keep the aggression issue current by, for example, putting it on the agenda at the annual unit review.

E Examine the environment. Ask whether the current facilities are likely to help or hinder the occurrence of aggression. Are you putting yourself at risk unnecessarily?

V Ventilate your concerns. Remember, if you feel frightened in certain situations, report it.

E Enlist the help of others. Talking to others can help to generate ideas and suggestions.

N Note the views of patients on how the facilities and staff behaviour might be improved. Get to know your patients' needs. The importance of developing a good nurse–patient relationship cannot be stressed too often.

T Tell new staff about the unit's aggression management policy. Teach and guide junior staff.

I Investigate and record all incidents. Ensure that you and your colleagues are familiar with the recording system.

O Observe the behaviour of others engaged in aggressive encounters. Use this as a learning experience to refine your own skills.

N Never be complacent: aggression can damage your health.

References

Abercrombie K (1968) Paralanguage. *British Journal of Communication*, **3**: 55–9.

Archer J (1967) The organisation of aggression and fear in vertebrates. In: Bateston P P G and Klopfer P (eds) *Perspectives in Ethology*, vol. 2. New York: Plenum Press.

Argyle M (1988) *Bodily Communication*, 2nd edn. London: Methuen.

Aronson E (1980) *The Social Animal*, 3rd edn. San Francisco: W H Freeman and Co.

Atkinson R L, Atkinson R C, Smith E C, Bem D J and Hilgard E R (1990) *Introduction to Psychology*, 10th edn. London: Harcourt, Brace and Jovanovich International.

Bandura A L (1973) *Aggression: A Social Learning Analysis.* New Jersey: Prentice Hall.

Baradell J G (1985) Humanistic care of the patient in seclusion. *Journal of Psychosocial Nursing*, **23**(2): 9–14.

Beckmann Murray R and Wilson Huelskoetter M M (1983) *Psychiatric/Mental Health Nursing: Giving Emotional Care.* New Jersey: Prentice Hall.

Berne E (1964) *Games People Play: the Psychology of Human Relationships.* Harmondsworth: Penguin.

Bolton R (1986) *People Skills: How To Assert Yourself, Listen To Others and Resolve Conflicts.* Sydney: Prentice Hall.

Brammer L M (1979) *The Helping Relationship: Process and Skills*, 2nd edn. New Jersey: Prentice Hall.

Breakwell G M (1989) *Facing Physical Violence.* London: British Psychological Society and Routledge.

Christie H and O'Reilly M (1984) Quality circles. *Nursing Mirror*, **158**(6): 16–19.

Confederation of Health Service Employees (1977) *The Management of Violent or Potentially Violent Patients.* Banstead: COHSE.

Dass R and Gorman P (1985) *How can I help?* London: Rider.

Department of Health (1989) *A Strategy for Nursing.* London: DoH.

Department of Health (1990a) *Code of Practice: Mental Health Act 1983*, p. 74. London: HMSO.

Department of Health (1990b) *Guidance for Clinical Health Care Workers: Protection Against Infection with HIV and Hepatitis Viruses.* London: HMSO.

DeVito, J A (1989) *The Interpersonal Communication Book*, 5th edn. New York: Harper and Row.

Di Bella C A (1979) Educating staff to manage threatening paranoid patients. *American Journal of Psychiatry*, **136**(3): 333–5.

Dickson D A, Hargie O and Morrow N C (1989) *Communication Skills Training for Health Professionals: An Instructor's Handbook.* London: Chapman and Hall.

Drummond D J, Sparr L F and Gordon G H (1989) Hospital violence reduction among high risk patients. *JAMA*, **261**(17): 2531–4.

Dusay J M (1977) *Egograms: How I See You and You See Me.* New York: Bantam Books.

Ekman P and Freisen W V (1969) Nonverbal leakage and cues to deception. *Psychiatry*, **32**: 88–106.

Ekman P, Freisen W V and Scherer K R (1976) Body movement and voice pitch in deceptive interaction. *Semiotica*, **16**: 233–7.

Farrell G A (1989) Responding to aggression: the role of significant others for student psychiatric nurses – an ethnographic study. *Nurse Education Today*, **9**: 335–40.

Feindler E L (1979) *Cognitive and Behavioural Approaches to Anger Control Training in Explosive Adolescents.* Unpublished doctoral dissertation, West Virginia University.

Feindler E L and Fremouw W J (1983) Stress inoculation training for adolescent anger problems pp. 451–485 in Chapter 13. In: Meichenbaum D and Jaremko M E (eds), *Stress Reduction and Prevention.* New York: Plenum Press.

Feindler E L, Marriott S A and Iwata M (1984) Group anger control training for junior high school delinquents. *Cognitive Therapy and Research*, **8**: 299–311.

Feindler E L, Latini J, Nape K, Romano J and Doyle J (1980) Anger reduction methods for child care workers at a residential delinquent facility. Presented at Association for the Advancement of Behaviour Therapy, New York City.

Feldman E, Mayou R, Hawton K, Arden M and Smith E B O (1987) Psychiatric disorder in medical in-patients. *Quarterly Journal of Medicine*, New Series, **241**: 405–12.

Finney G (1988) One false move. *Community Outlook*, **April**: 8–9.

Freud S (1905) Fragments of an analysis of a case of hysteria. Reprinted in Strachey J (ed.), 1953, *The Standard Edition of the Complete Psychological Works of Sigmund Freud*, vol. 7, p. 78. London: Hogarth Press.

Fried M L and DeFazio V J (1974) Territoriality and boundary conflicts in the subway. *Psychiatry*, **34**: 47–59.

Frost M (1974) *Nursing Care of the Schizophrenic Patient.* London: Henry Kimpton.

Gerry E M (1989) An investigation into the assertive behaviour of trained nurses in general hospital settings. *Journal of Advanced Nursing*, **14**: 1002–8.

Gibson B (1989) The use of seclusion. *Nursing*, **33**(43): 24–6.

Gillespie V and Orton A (1985) Watching while you wait. *Nursing Times*, **81** (39): 40–2.

Goldstein A P and Keller H (1987) *Aggressive Behaviour: Assessment and Intervention.* Exeter: Pergamon.

Gorski T T and Miller M (1986) *The Management of Aggression and Violence.* San Francisco: Herald House.

Gostin L (1986) *Institutions Observed.* London, King Edward's Hospital Fund for London.

Hall E T (1959) *The Silent Language.* New York: Doubleday.

Hall J (1988) Unpublished report. Top Grade Psychologist, Warneford Hospital, Warneford Lane, Oxford.

Haller M and Deluty R H (1988) Assaults on staff by psychiatric in-patients: a critical review. *British Journal of Psychiatry*, **152**: 174–9.

Hargie O, Saunders C and Dickson D (1987) *Social Skills in Interpersonal Communication.* London: Routledge.

Health Services Advisory Committee (1987) *Violence to Staff in the Health Services.* London: HMSO.

Horowitz M J, Duff D F and Stratton L O (1964) Body buffer zone. *Archives of General Psychiatry*, **11**: 651–6.

Kaplan S G and Wheeler E G (1983) Survival skills for working with potentially violent clients. *Social Casework*, **64**: 334–46.

Janis I L (1958) *Psychological Stress*. New York: Wiley.

Kinzel A S (1970) Body buffer zone in violent prisoners. *American Journal of Psychiatry*, **127**: 59–64.

Kitson A (1990) *Quality Patient Care: The Dynamic Standard Setting System*. London: Scutari Press.

Klama J (1988) *Aggression: Conflict in Animals and Humans Reconsidered*. Essex: Longman Scientific and Technical.

Kornfeld D S (1969) Psychiatric view of the intensive care unit. *British Medical Journal*, **1**: 108–10.

Lange S P (1978) *Behavioural Concepts and Nursing Interventions*, 2nd edn. Philadelphia: Lippincott.

Lanza M L (1983) The reactions of nursing staff to physical assault by a patient. *Hospital and Community Psychiatry*, **34**: 44–7.

Lanza M L (1984) A follow-up study of nurses' reactions to physical assault. *Hospital and Community Psychiatry*, **35**: 492–4.

Lowe T (1990) *Challenging Behaviour*. Unpublished report. Littlemore Hospital, Littlemore, Oxford.

Lucas M J and Folstein (1980) Nursing assessment of mental disorders on a general medical unit. *Journal of Psychiatric Nursing*, **18**: 31–3.

Lyttle J (1986) *Mental Disorder: Its Care and Treatment*. London: Baillière Tindall.

Martin J P (1984) *Hospitals in Trouble*. London: Blackwell.

Mental Health Act (1983) London: HMSO.

Minot S R and Adamski T J (1989) Elements of effective clinical supervision. *Perspectives in Psychiatric Care*, **25**(2): 22–6.

Morris D (1977) *Manwatching: A Field Guide to Human Behaviour*. London: Jonathan Cape.

Nelson-Jones R (1988) *Practical Counselling and Helping Skills*, 2nd edn. London: Cassell.

Nichols K A (1984) *Psychological Care in Physical Illness*. London: Croom Helm.

Ohbuchi K, Kameda M and Agarie N (1989) Apology as aggression control: its role in mediating appraisal of and response to harm. *Journal of Personality and Social Psychology*, **56**(2): 219–27.

Oreschnik R (1984) Quality of care. *Senior Nurse*, **1**(16): 13–15.

Pearson M and Smith D (1985) Debriefing in experience-based learning. In: Boud D, Keogh R and Walker D, *Reflection: Turning Experience into Learning*, pp. 69–84. London: Kogan Page.

Platt-Koch L M (1986) Clinical supervision for psychiatric nurses. *Journal of Psychosocial Nursing*, **26**(1): 7–15.

Reber A S (1985) *The Penguin Dictionary of Psychology*. Harmondsworth: Penguin.

Robson M (1984) *Quality Circles in Action*. London: Gower.

Rosenhan D L (1973) On being sane in insane places. *Science*, **179**: 250–8.

Rosenthal R (1964) Experimental outcome-orientation and the results of the psychological experiment. *Psychological Bulletin*, **61**: 405–12.

Royal College of Nursing (1979) *Seclusion and Restraint in Hospitals and Units for the Mentally Disordered*. London: RCN.

Royal College of Nursing (1985) *Nursing Guidelines on the Management of Patients in Hospital and in the Community Suffering from AIDS*. London: RCN.

Royal College of Nursing (1987) *Focus on Restraint*. London: RCN.

Salkovskis P M (1989) Somatic problems. In: Hawton K, Salkovskis P M, Kirk J and Clark D M, *Cognitive Behaviour Therapy for Psychiatric Problems: A practical Guide*, pp. 235–274. Oxford: Oxford University Press.

Salmon P and Farrell G (1983) The long stay psychiatric patient. *Nursing Times,* **79** (issue no. 37): 89–40.

Schachter S and Singer (1962) Cognitive, social and psychological determinants of emotional state. *Psychological Review,* **69**: 379–99.

Schon D A (1983) *The Reflective Practitioner: How Professionals Think in Action.* New York: Basic Books.

Sieff M (1990) *On Management.* London: Weidenfeld and Nicolson.

Simpson I H, Back K, Ingles T, Kerckhoff A and McKinney J C (1979) *From Student to Nurse: A Longitudinal Study of Socialisation.* Cambridge: Cambridge University Press.

Smith A and Russell J (1991) Using critical learning incidents in nurse education. *Nurse Education Today,* **11**: 284–91.

Smith M (1975) *When I Say No I Feel Guilty.* London: Bantam Books.

Stedeford A (1983) *Facing Death.* London: Heinemann.

Steiner C M (1970) A fairytale. *Transactional Analysis Journal,* **9**(36): 146.

Stockwell F C (1972) *The Unpopular Patient.* London: RCN.

Stuart G W and Sundeen S J (1983) *Principles and Practice of Psychiatric Nursing.* St Louis: C V Mosby.

Sugden J (1985) Labelling theory. *Nursing* (Second Series), Vol. 2, no. 35 p. 1021. Oxford.

Swanson H (1976) The biological value of aggression. In: Tutt N (ed.), *Violence,* pp. 338–345. London: HMSO.

Thompson D R (1989) A randomised controlled trial of in-hospital nursing support for first time myocardial infarction patients and their partners: effects on anxiety and depression. *Journal of Advanced Nursing,* **14**: 291–7.

Trades Union Congress (1988) *Hazards at Work: TUC Guide to Health and Safety.* London: TUC.

Travelbee J (1976) *Interpersonal Aspects of Nursing.* Philadelphia: F A Davis.

Tupin T (1975) Management of violent patients. In: Shader R (ed.), *Manual of Psychiatric Therapeutics,* chapter 7. Boston: Little Brown and Co.

United Kingdom Central Council for Nursing, Midwifery and Health Visiting (1984) *Code of Conduct.* London: UKCC.

United Kingdom Central Council for Nursing, Midwifery and Health Visiting (1990). Report of the Post-Registration Education and Practice Project. London: UKCC.

Volicer B J and Bohannon M W (1974) Patients' perceptions of stressful events associated with hospitalisation. *Nursing Research,* **23**, May–June: 235–8.

Walton M (1984) *Management and Managing: A Dynamic Approach.* London: Harper and Row.

Wiener H (1979) Human exocrinology: the olfactory component of nonverbal communication. In: Weitz S (ed.), *Nonverbal Communication,* 2nd edn. New York: Oxford University Press.

Weitz S (1979) *Nonverbal Communication,* 2nd edn. New York: Oxford University Press.

Whittington R and Wykes T (1989) Invisible injury. *Nursing Times,* **85**(42): 30–2.

Whittington R and Wykes T (1992) Staff strain and social support in a psychiatric hospital following assault by a patient. *Journal of Advanced Nursing,* **17**: 480–6.

Wondrak R (1989) Dealing with verbal abuse. *Nurse Education Today,* **9**: 276–80.

Woodward T (1989) Personal Communication. Charge Nurse, Phoenix Unit, Littlemore Hospital, Littlemore, Oxford.

Wright B (1989) Threatening behaviour. *Nursing Times,* **85**(42): 26–9.

Index